T0215050

Lao She's *Teahouse* and Its Two English Translations

Lao She's Teahouse *and Its Two English Translations: Exploring Chinese Drama Translation with Systemic Functional Linguistics* provides an in-depth application of Systemic Functional Linguistics (SFL) to the study of Chinese drama translation and theoretically explores the interface between SFL and drama translation.

Investigating two English translations of the Chinese drama *Teahouse* (茶馆 *Cha Guan* in Chinese) by Lao She, and translated by John Howard-Gibbon and Ying Ruocheng respectively, Bo Wang and Yuanyi Ma apply Systemic Functional Linguistics to point out the choices that translators have to make in translation.

This book is of interest to graduates and researchers of Chinese translation and discourse studies.

Bo Wang and **Yuanyi Ma** received their doctoral degrees from the Hong Kong Polytechnic University. Their research interests include Systemic Functional Linguistics, translation studies, discourse analysis, and language description. They are co-authors of *Systemic Functional Translation Studies: Theoretical Insights and New Directions*, *Translating Tagore's* Stray Birds *into Chinese: Applying Systemic Functional Linguistics to Chinese Poetry Translation* and *Systemic Functional Insights on Language and Linguistics*. Bo Wang is currently Associate Research Fellow at the School of International Studies, Sun Yat-sen University, China. Yuanyi Ma is Lecturer at Guangdong Polytechnic of Science and Technology, China.

Routledge Studies in Chinese Translation

Series Editor: Chris Shei

Swansea University, UK

This series encompasses scholarly works on every possible translation activity and theory involving the use of Chinese language. Putting together an important knowledge base for Chinese and Westerner researchers on translation studies, the series draws on multiple disciplines for essential information and further research that is based on or relevant to Chinese translation.

For more information about this series, please visit: www.routledge.com/languages/series/RSCT

Lao She's *Teahouse* and Its Two English Translations

Exploring Chinese Drama Translation with Systemic Functional Linguistics

Bo Wang and Yuanyi Ma

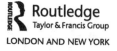

Routledge
Taylor & Francis Group

LONDON AND NEW YORK

First published 2020
by Routledge
2 Park Square, Milton Park, Abingdon, Oxon OX14 4RN

and by Routledge
52 Vanderbilt Avenue, New York, NY 10017

Routledge is an imprint of the Taylor & Francis Group, an informa business

British Library Cataloguing-in-Publication Data
A catalogue record for this book is available from the British Library

Library of Congress Cataloging-in-Publication Data
Names: Wang, Bo, (Professor of translation studies), author. | Ma, Yuanyi, author.
Title: Lao She's Teahouse and its two English translations : exploring
  Chinese drama translation with systemic functional linguistics/Bo Wang,
  Yuanyi Ma.
Description: London; New York : Routledge, 2020. | Series: Routledge studies
  in Chinese translation | Includes bibliographical references and index.
Identifiers: LCCN 2019054042 (print) | LCCN 2019054043 (ebook) |
  ISBN 9780367261887 (hardback) | ISBN 9780367261917 (paperback) |
  ISBN 9780429291920 (ebook)
Subjects: LCSH: Lao, She, 1899–1966. Cha guan. | Lao, She, 1899–1966 –
  Translations into English – History and criticism. | Chinese drama –
  Translations into English – History and criticism. | Chinese language –
  Translating into English. | Translating and interpreting.
Classification: LCC PL2804.C5 C5375 2020 (print) | LCC PL2804.C5 (ebook) |
  DDC 428/.0420951 – dc23
LC record available at https://lccn.loc.gov/2019054042
LC ebook record available at https://lccn.loc.gov/2019054043

ISBN: 978-0-367-26188-7 (hbk)
ISBN: 978-0-367-26191-7 (pbk)
ISBN: 978-0-429-29192-0 (ebk)

Typeset in Times New Roman
by Apex CoVantage, LLC

Contents

Figures

Tables

Foreword

This book is a welcome addition to the literature on systemic functionally informed translation studies. It sets out to apply Systemic Functional Linguistics to the analysis of two English translations of the Chinese playscript of *Teahouse*, which consists of three types of text: dramatic dialogue, dramatic monologue, and stage direction. The authors have developed their own analytical framework for the linguistic analysis and comparison of the original and its translations. This analytical framework has proved to be adequate for explaining exactly how the translations of *Teahouse* function in their contexts of situation and their contexts of culture. The framework was shown to facilitate the close analysis of the choices made by the translators in the playscript's three types of texts, i.e. choices in the systems of MOOD, THEME, TAXIS, and LOGICO-SEMANTIC TYPE.

The analytical system used by the authors also made it possible to identify, quantify, and discuss the metafunctional translation shift. These shifts could be explained with reference to a crucial – although in nonlinguistic circles often misunderstood and denigrated – notion in translation theory: equivalence. To achieve equivalence in the face of typological differences between the language pair involved in the translations on hand, translators needed to conduct shifts on different linguistic levels and dimensions. Thanks to the analytic instrumentarium provided by Systemic Functional Linguistics, it was possible to discover, name, classify, and explain such translational shifts.

This is an excellent and innovative book that shows how useful Systemic Functional Linguistics is in analyzing, comparing, and evaluating translations. The framework proposed here can be fruitfully used with different language pairs by linguists and translation scholars across the world who are interested in linguistically analyzing translators' choices and translators' styles with the help of an approach most appropriate for translation studies.

The work presented in this book also has important implications for typological studies and investigations of translation universals.

I congratulate the two young translation scholars for their innovative work, and I trust that readers of this book will join me in this praise.

Juliane House

Preface

This is a book written for researchers and students who wish to apply Systemic Functional Linguistics (SFL) to translation studies in general and drama translation in particular. In this book, we explain the important concepts used in our analysis and would like to encourage our readers to carry out their own text analysis after reading the book. Also, for the convenience of readers who do not know Mandarin Chinese, we provide pinyin, interlinear glossing, and back translation for the examples throughout the book.

This is a book that aims to illuminate translation as a linguistic process, to apply SFL to drama translation, and to explore the relationship between theory and evidences. The book investigates a Chinese drama entitled *Teahouse* (茶馆 *Cha Guan* in Chinese) written by Lao She, and its two English translations by John Howard-Gibbon and Ying Ruocheng. Six chapters are included in the book.

Chapter 1 orients the study in SFL and translation studies by briefly introducing the background of SFL and its applications to translation. In addition, the data of the present study is introduced, with three kinds of text being identified, i.e. dramatic dialogue, dramatic monologue, and stage direction. An analytical framework that considers the three kinds of text and involves different systems of language is constructed based on a preliminary analysis.

Chapter 2 reports on the interpersonal analysis of mood choices in the dramatic dialogue. The analysis is further related to the characterization of the leading characters in *Teahouse* and some patterns of changes in mood type are found in the target texts (TTs). **Chapter 3** and **Chapter 4** focus on the textual and the logical mode of meanings respectively. Chapter 3 explores the textual choices in the system of THEME in dramatic monologue, and Chapter 4 investigates the logical choices in the systems of TAXIS and LOGICO-SEMANTIC TYPE in stage direction. Moreover, from Chapter 2 to Chapter 4, various types of metafunctional translation shifts are examined, which are shifts that appear within one and the same metafunction, viz. mood shift, Theme shift, tactic shift, and logico-semantic type shift.

Chapter 5 examines the data from the perspectives of the three contextual parameters, i.e. field, tenor, and mode, and points out the similarities and differences between the source text and the two target texts in terms of these parameters. Contextual analysis has provided some evidence for the lexicogrammatical choices discussed in Chapters 2, 3, and 4, because the translators' choices are to some extent influenced by context.

Chapter 6 synthesizes the major findings from Chapter 2 to Chapter 5. It also summarizes the contributions of the book in terms of (i) the appliability of SFL theory, (ii) the development of "the environments of translation" and "metafunctional translation shift" proposed by Matthiessen (2001, 2014b), (iii) the validity of the analytical framework proposed, (iv) the implications for translation practice and typological studies, and (v) the investigations of translation universals. This chapter also recommends some directions for future research.

Acknowledgments

We would like to express our heartfelt thanks to Professor Christian M.I.M. Matthiessen, who opened the door of SFL for us, enriches our understandings of linguistics, and continues to inspire us along our academic path.

We thank Professor Juliane House for her warm support all along and for kindly writing a Foreword for this book.

We also extend our thanks to people who helped and encouraged us during the process of writing this book, including Professor Chu Chi-yu, Dr. Chris Shei, Dr. Constance Wang, Professor Erich Steiner, Professor Huang Guowen, Professor Chang Chenguang, Dr. Marvin Lam, Dr. Elaine Espindola, Dr. Lise Fontaine, Dr. Jorge Arús-Hita, and Dr. Isaac Mwinlaaru.

Our special thanks goes to Dr. Mark Nartey for proofreading the draft of this book.

Abbreviations and symbols

BT	back translation
IG	interlinear glossing
PY	pinyin
RST	Rhetorical Structure Theory
SFL	Systemic Functional Linguistics
SFTS	systemic functional translation studies
ST	source text
TT	target text
TT1	target text 1 – John Howard-Gibbon's translation (Lao 2004)
TT2	target text 2 – Ying Ruocheng's translation (Lao 1999)
↘	realization
∕	conflation
^	ordering (followed by)
< >	enclosed group/phrase
<< >>	enclosed clause
<<< >>>	enclosed clause complex
ø	ellipsis
‖‖	clause complex, boundary markers
‖	clause (not rankshifted), boundary markers
		phrase or group, boundary markers
[[[ ]]]	rankshifted (embedded) clause complex, boundary markers
[[ ]]	rankshifted (embedded) clause, boundary markers
[]	rankshifted group/phrase, boundary markers
α	and other small Greek letters: elements of hypotactic interdependency structure
1	and other Arabic numerals: elements of paratactic interdependency structure
+	logico-semantic relation of extension
=	logico-semantic relation of elaboration
×	logico-semantic relation of enhancement
'	projection of idea
"	projection of locution
//	line break

Abbreviations for interlinear glossing

APART	adverbial particle
ASP	clause particle: aspectual
CV	coverb
DISP	voice coverb: dispositive
EMPH	emphatic
HON	honorific
MEAS	measurer
MOD	verbal particle: modal
NEG	verbal particle: negative
PV	postverb
SUB	subordinating
VADV	verbal adverb
VPART	verbal particle

1 Mapping and approaching Systemic Functional Linguistics and translation

In this chapter, we first situate the present study in Systemic Functional Linguistics (SFL) by introducing the historical background and the status quo of applying SFL to translation in Section 1.1. In Section 1.2, we offer a brief account of *Teahouse* (茶馆), a Chinese drama written by Lao She, which is regarded as monumental work in the history of Chinese literature. We then discuss our classification of the three kinds of text in *Teahouse*. Section 1.3 presents the research methods, elaborates on the analytical framework, and discusses the data size.

1.1 Systemic Functional Linguistics and translation

The past 50 years have witnessed the rapid development of Systemic Functional Linguistics (SFL), a theory that approaches language from various dimensions and understands language in context rather than in isolation (see Halliday 1985a, 1994a; Halliday & Matthiessen 2004, 2014 for SFL descriptions of English grammar). Unlike Chomsky's (e.g. 1957, 1965, 2006) formal approach to language, according to which theory is isolated from application, SFL is an appliable theory that is not only designed to be applied but also remains in constant dialogue with application (Halliday 1985b, 2008; Matthiessen 2014a). This distinction between the functional approach to language and the formal approach is characterized as "ecologism" versus "formalism" in Seuren (1998) or "language as resource" versus "language as rule" in Halliday (1977).

Halliday (1964, 1985b) regards his theory of language as essentially consumer-oriented and admits that the value of a theory lies in its application. Consequently, SFL has been applied to different areas of language sciences including translation (Matthiessen 2009; see Wang & Ma in press for a detailed survey of this area). Systemic functional linguists view translation as a relation between languages, as a process of moving from one language to another, and as recreation of meaning in context. Halliday (2009) regards translation as a specialized domain, because relatively few formal or functional linguists have paid explicit attention to translation. He also recognizes translation as a kind of testing ground, and argues that a theory is inadequate if it "cannot account for the phenomenon of translation" (ibid.: 17). One prerequisite for applying SFL to translation is that SFL provides a theoretical basis of language description, with English, Chinese and various

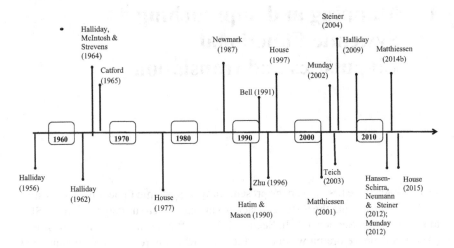

Figure 1.1 A timeline of some important studies that apply SFL to translation

languages being described from the SFL perspective (e.g. Caffarel, Martin & Matthiessen 2004; Martin, Doran & Figueredo 2019; see Mwinlaaru & Xuan 2016 for an overview of this area).

The origin of applying SFL to translation, according to Steiner (2005, 2015, 2019), can be traced to the early British contextualism, i.e. Malinowski's (e.g. 1923, 1935) anthropological studies on context and translation on the Trobriand Islands in Papua New Guinea. Malinowski (1935) emphasizes the role that translation plays in understanding an aboriginal language. He holds that translation is crucial in bringing out the differences between the meanings in some other cultures and his own English-speaking culture. Different from the missionary linguists' Eurocentric view of translation that tries to assimilate the foreign culture into the target culture, Malinowski's approach (1935) acknowledges the role that the context of culture plays by recognizing the differences between the source culture and the target culture. Malinowski's (e.g. 1923, 1935) notion of context was inherited by Firth, who influenced Halliday and SFL.

Figure 1.1 is a timeline that highlights some important studies of applying SFL to translation, reflecting the chronological development of theorizing and modeling translation from the SFL perspective. In accordance with Halliday's (2001) characterization of translation theories, these studies in the timeline are descriptive rather than prescriptive, and can be considered as linguists' theories of translation rather than those of translators.

1.1.1   *Early studies before the 1970s*

Translation has been on the agenda of SFL since the 1950s, marked by Halliday's (1956, 1962) engagement with machine translation in his early career. Halliday

(1956) highlights the importance of linguistic analysis, states the futility of one-to-one translation equivalent, and emphasizes the need for describing the languages involved in machine translation. In this work, we find the initial ideas of SFL, such as (i) the paradigmatic organization in language description by regarding lexis as a resource and (ii) the notion of making choices in a thesaurus, which is capable of providing the different options available and is different from a dictionary. In his next paper on machine translation, Halliday (1962) applies his scale and category theory to machine translation, involving the grammatical categories of "level," "unit," "structure," "form," and "rank." He relates translation equivalence to the rank scale of lexicogrammar, and distinguishes three steps in the process of translation:

> First, there is the selection of the "most probable translation equivalent" for each item at each rank, based on simple frequency. Second, there is the conditioning effect of the surrounding text in the source language on these probabilities: here grammatical and lexical features of the unit next above are taken into account and may (or may not) lead to the choice of an item other than the one with highest overall probability. Third, there is the internal structure of the target language, which may (or may not) lead to the choice of yet another item as a result of grammatical and lexical relations particular to that language: these can be viewed as brought into operation similarly by step-by-step progression up the rank scale.
>
> (Halliday 1962: 153)

A follow-up work in this area is the chapter titled "Comparison and Translation" by Halliday, McIntosh and Strevens (1964), in which they discuss the relationship between language comparison, translation, and language teaching. They ground translation in language description and comparison, which include the following three steps: (i) the separate description of related features of each language, (ii) the establishment of comparability, and (iii) the comparison itself. Also, they apply the linguistic descriptions of stratum and rank in translation. Figure 1.2 shows how translation equivalence can be maintained at different ranks of

Translation at rank of:	||| elle	se	frott+a+			les +		joue +s	
morpheme	X	X	rub	X	X	X	X	cheek	X
word	she/her	X	rubbed			the		cheeks	
group	she	rubbed			herself	his/her		cheeks	
clause	she	rubbed				her		cheeks	

Figure 1.2 Multilingual correspondence and rank

Source: Adapted from Halliday, McIntosh & Strevens (1964: 127)

lexicogrammar when translating from French to English. At the clause rank, translation equivalence is the easiest to achieve; thus, it is appropriate to translate the clause in French into one in English, as the clause rank is the widest grammatical environment where the text is maximally contextualized and where there is a higher degree of grammatically specified translation equivalence (see Matthiessen 2001). By contrast, at the rank of morpheme, equivalence is the most difficult to achieve, with only equivalent choices of two French morphemes – "frott" and "joue" being found in English. However, by moving upward along the rank scale from morpheme to clause, we find more equivalent choices between the two languages.

The overall application continues with Catford (1965), who formulates a general theory of translation based on Halliday's (1961) scale and category grammar – an early version of systemic functional grammar. In Catford's (1965) monograph, translation equivalence and translation shift are examined from the perspectives of rank and stratification (termed as level, which include context, form: grammar and lexis, and substance: graphology or phonology). Catford (1965) takes the search of translation equivalents in the target language as the crucial issue of translation practice and regards the nature and conditions of translation equivalence as the critical task of translation theory.

1.1.2 Studies from the 1970s to the millennium

From the late 1960s to 1980s, Halliday (1961) increasingly focuses on the paradigmatic system, thus treating the syntagmatic structure as the realization of the choices made in the system. Semantics, along with lexicogrammar, is considered as a stratum of the content plane. Also, the three metafunctions, i.e. the ideational, the interpersonal, and the textual, are identified and dealt with at the level of semantics and lexicogrammar (Halliday 1967a, 1967b, 1985b). Along with the developments in SFL, House (1977) proposes her model of translation quality assessment during the latter half of the 1970s. Based on the equivalence between the source text and the target text, her model remains one of the most influential frameworks to translation criticism. Conceiving translation as recontextualization, House's (e.g. 1977, 1997, 2015) model heavily depends on the Hallidayan analysis of field, tenor, and mode. Lexicogrammatical analysis is also incorporated, which is regarded as realizations of register and genre. House's model provides theoretical motivations for two translation strategies, i.e. overt translation and covert translation. The concept of the cultural filter, which captures the sociocultural differences, is also highlighted.

Since the 1980s, the appliability of SFL has been widely recognized in translation studies (e.g. Newmark 1987; Taylor 1993; Munday 2001; Steiner 2005, 2015). Different aspects of SFL have shed light on a number of studies. For instance, some researches are oriented toward the stratum of semantics. Hatim and Mason (1990) consider translation at the stratum of semantics, adopting the SFL concepts of genre, register, and cohesion to examine translation equivalence on lexical, grammatical, textual, and pragmatic levels. Bell (1991) demonstrates the significance of a linguistic theory to translation by proposing a model of translation both as process and as product based on SFL. Zhu (1996) constructs his model of structure of meaning by integrating SFL with Austin's (1962) speech act theory.

1.1.3 Studies after the millennium

The 2000s have witnessed a renewed interest in applying SFL to translation, marked by the publication of *Exploring Translation and Multilingual Text Production: Beyond Content* edited by Steiner and Yallop (2001) – most chapters in this book are informed by SFL. It is noteworthy that Halliday (2001, 2009, 2010) also has several publications on SFL and translation in this period. These studies characterize translation theories, introduce the theoretical approaches, emphasize the notion of making choices in translation, and illustrate how SFL can be applied to translation.

Some studies after the millennium are characterized by the integration of corpus-based methodology and SFL analysis. On the one hand, corpora can trigger studies on a range of topics. For instance, the corpora built by Steiner and his research team in Saarbrücken – CroCo (Crosslinguistic Corpora for Translation) (Hansen-Schirra, Neumann & Steiner 2012) provided resources for studies on explicitation in translation (Steiner 2008), translation of grammatical metaphor (Steiner 2002), and comparison of cohesion between German and English (Steiner 2017). On the other hand, there are also frameworks that incorporate corpus methodology, such as Munday's (2002) attempt of combining SFL, corpus linguistics, and the analysis of the cultural and the social context.

Moreover, some studies after the noughts (e.g. Matthiessen 2001; Teich 2001, 2003) have become increasingly comprehensive, which represent "a movement of theorizing along the stratification dimension" (Steiner 2005: 487). For example, Matthiessen (2001) contextualizes translation and locates it within a typology of systems, which he names as "the environments of translation," i.e. what translators have access to that informs their choices in translation. By following this approach, translation has for the first time been studied within an overall SFL-architecture. Matthiessen (2001) proposes six dimensions, which together define the environments of translation, including stratification, instantiation, rank, metafunction, delicacy, and axis. Figure 1.2 illustrates the dimension of rank scale in lexicogrammar, according to which clause is the widest environment and morpheme is the narrowest environment. Similarly, the notion of rank scale can be applied to other dimensions, and the amount of information available to translators depends on the environment they have access to. Therefore, in "literal" translation, translators have access to the narrow grammatical environment of the text in this context of situation; whereas in "free" translation, translators have access to the wide environment (see Figure 1.3). According to Matthiessen (2001: 74–75), the general principle is that "the wider the environment of translation, the higher the degree

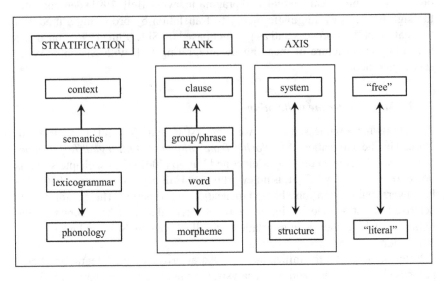

Figure 1.3 The environments and nature of translation
Source: Adapted from Matthiessen (2001: 81)

of translation equivalence." We can also note that in the "widest" environment, the text is "maximally contextualized," and is very likely to be "maximally effective" (Halliday 2010: 16). The principle can be formulated from an ecological perspective as follows:

> the higher the unit that you translate in terms of (i) stratification and (ii) within a given stratum, the more information you will have access to in order to make an informed choice.
>
> (Matthiessen forthcoming: 12)

In a follow-up study, Matthiessen (2014b) focuses on metafunction – one of the six dimensions. Translation is conceived as recreation of meaning in context through choice and "an ongoing process of choosing options within the systems of the source language and of the target language" (2014b: 272). Drawing on the four metafunctional modes of meaning, translation involves the recreation of ideational meanings of the logical kind, ideational meanings of the experiential kind, interpersonal meanings, and textual meanings. As shown in Figure 1.4, the different modes of meaning are identified by way of metafunctional analysis, which functions like a prism that identifies the various colors of white light (Matthiessen 2014b: 277, original emphasis):

> In terms of **logical** meaning, translators choose how to interpret logico-semantic relations used in forming "coherent" source texts, and they choose among

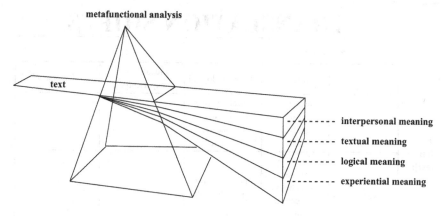

Figure 1.4 Modes of meaning in text revealed by the metafunctional part of discourse analysis

Source: Adapted from Matthiessen (2014b: 277)

the options in the target language to **reconstrue** them in the translation they are producing.

In terms of **experiential** meaning, translators choose how to interpret events as configurations of elements (processes, participants and circumstances) and larger "chunks" of experience made up of events such as episodes and procedures, and they choose among the options in the target language to **reconstrue** the experiential meanings in the translation they are producing.

In terms of **interpersonal** meaning, translators choose how to interpret propositions, proposals and the assessments associated with them in the exchange of meaning embodied in the source text, and they choose among the options in the target language to **reenact** the interpersonal meanings in the translation they are producing.

In terms of **textual** meaning, translators choose how to interpret messages and the sequences of messages that create the flow of information in the source text, and they choose among the options in the target language to **represent** the textual meanings in the translation they are producing.

Even though the four modes of meaning are equally implicated in language, they have not received equal attention in translation practice. The experiential meaning has primarily been the focus of the translators, while the textual meaning tends to be ignored in translation practice (Kim & Matthiessen 2015). In research, however, we can choose to analyze all the four modes of meaning or focus on one or several of them. For example, Kim and Huang (2012) investigate textual meaning by examining the professional translators' choices of Theme in three translations of a Chinese short story. Munday (2012, 2018) approaches the interpersonal meaning

TRANSLATION SHIFTS

From [source text]:

		textual	ideational: logical	ideational: experiential	interpersonal
To [target text]:	textual	textual > textual: e.g. theme shift	logical > textual: e.g. complex to cohesive sequence		
	ideational: logical	textual > logical: e.g. cohesive sequence to complex	logical > logical: e.g. tactic shift		
	ideational: experiential		logical > experiential: e.g. clause > phrase	experiential > experiential: e.g. process type shift	
	interpersonal				interpersonal > interpersonal: e.g. mood type shift

Figure 1.5 Matrix of metafunctional translation shifts
Source: Adapted from Matthiessen (2014b: 284)

by adopting Martin and White's (2005) appraisal framework. In this book, we cover three metafunctional modes of meaning, including the interpersonal (Chapter 2), the textual (Chapter 3), and the ideational meaning of the logical kind (Chapter 4).

The analysis that involves different metafunctional modes of meaning can be used to examine translation equivalence and translation shift. Matthiessen (2014b) provides one way of probing metafunctional translation shifts by categorizing them into general classes of choice in accordance with the four metafunctions (see Figure 1.5). This book deals with three kinds of metafunctional translation shift, namely shift from interpersonal to interpersonal (mood shift in Chapter 2), shift from textual to textual (Theme shift in Chapter 3), and shift from logical to logical (tactic shift and logico-semantic type shift in Chapter 4).

Alternatively, one can explore different text types or registers by using an SFL analysis. For instance, seminal studies on advertisements have been conducted by Steiner (2004) to examine the translations and registerial variation of the advertisements of Rolex watches. Yu and Wu (e.g. 2016, 2017) analyze *The Platform Sutra*, a collection of Master Huineng's personal conversations and public sermons from different perspectives. Huang (2006) selects ancient Chinese poems and lyrics as data in his pioneering analysis. In this book, our data include a play written in

Chinese and its two English translations, which are literary texts in the first place. Also, we categorize the playscript into three text types and analyze them differently. In the next section, we provide a brief account of the different kinds of text in *Teahouse*.

1.2   Three kinds of text in Lao She's *Teahouse*

Teahouse, the source text (ST) of the present study, is a drama written in Mandarin Chinese by Lao She – one of the most significant figures of 20th-century Chinese literature. First staged in 1958 by Beijing People's Art Theatre, it is regarded as a monumental work in the history of Chinese drama and is famous for its vivid depiction of characters (Cao 2007). As Lao She's most representative drama written after the founding of the People's Republic of China, *Teahouse* presents three splendid episodes of modern Chinese history, i.e. the late Qing Dynasty in 1898, the early Republic of China under the warlords' reign in 1917, and the period following the defeat of the Japanese in 1945. All three acts of the play take place in the same teahouse, achieving one kind of special unity. Further, *Teahouse* does not solely rely on one major character to weave its plot but rather involves a huge cast of around 70 characters from all walks of life in Chinese society, such as the manager of the teahouse, eunuch, fortune-teller, Manchurian customer, secret police, peasant, gangster, and modern businessman (Tam 2004). By portraying the life of these characters, Lao She gives us a panoramic view of the Chinese nation and its people.

The data in the present study also include two English translations of the play, one by John Howard-Gibbon (target text 1, TT1) (Lao 1980, 2004) and the other by Ying Ruocheng (target text 2, TT2) (Lao 1999, 2003). Previous studies have noted that the two translators render this drama with different purposes: TT1 is translated to be read, while TT2 is translated to be performed on stage. Also, various changes have been made in TT2 by the translator for purposes of performability (e.g. Ren 2008; Yang 2016; Wang 2017).

In this book, we attempt to categorize the playscript of *Teahouse* into three kinds of text, namely dramatic dialogue, dramatic monologue, and stage direction (see Figure 1.6). Of the three, dramatic dialogue constitutes the major part of the play, while dramatic monologue and stage direction are largely supportive. However, unlike previous studies, which tend to focus only on dramatic dialogue (e.g. Ren 2008), we take all three kinds of text into consideration, trying to obtain a complete picture of the language of the play.

Dramatic dialogue, as the major concern of the playwrights, is referred to as the "speech between two or more characters that conveys information or tone to the audience" (Kennedy 2010: 166) and is normally regarded as one of the basic components of a playscript, along with stage direction. *Teahouse* includes a large amount of dramatic dialogue in which we find abundant use of satire and humor – "two things that Lao She learned from Western literature, particularly from the comedies by the Great dramatist Aristophanes" (Tam 2004: xliv; cf. Lao 1982). As shown in Example 1.1, the sarcastic language in Tang the Oracle's line helps to

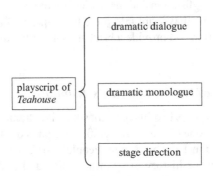

Figure 1.6 Three kinds of text in *Teahouse*

portray a shameless drug addict who considers taking drugs as pleasure (see Sections 2.2.9 and 5.2.2.2).

Example 1.1 (adapted from Lao 1999: 78–79, 2004: 68–69)

ST: 大英帝国 的 烟，日本的 "白面儿"，两 大 强 国 伺候 着 我一个人，这点 福气 还 小 吗?

PY: dà yīng dì guó de yān, rì běn de "bái miàn er," liǎng dà qiáng guó cì hou zhe wǒ yí gè rén, zhèi diǎn fú qì hái xiǎo ma

IG: British Empire SUB cigarette, Japanese heroin, two great powerful nation look after VPART myself, this good fortune EMPH small MOD

BT: British Empire's cigarettes and Japanese heroin, two great powerful nations look after myself. Isn't that very good fortune?

TT1: British Imperial Cigarettes and Japanese heroin – I'm being looked after by the big boys. Now, wouldn't you call that good fortune?

TT2: British imperial cigarettes and Japanese heroin! Two great powers looking after poor little me. Aren't I lucky?

In addition, the dramatic dialogue in *Teahouse* is characterized by the use of Beijing dialect. For instance, the lexical choice of "甭" (PY: béng; IG: do not) – a combination of "不 用" (PY: bú yòng; IG: NEG need) in Example 1.2 can be seen in northern dialects in China (including Beijing dialect) and is seldom found in daily conversations of people from Guangdong Province in the southern part of China.

Example 1.2 (adapted from Lao 1999: 38–39, 2004: 38–39)

ST: 你 甭 再 耍 无赖，不 长 房钱!

PY: nǐ béng zài shuǎ wú lài, bù zhǎng fáng qián

IG: you do not again play trick, NEG raise rent

BT: Don't play tricks again, and do not raise the rent!

TT1: Don't give me any more of your tripe about not raising the rent.

TT2: Don't you dare play your tricks and refuse to raise the rent!

In the dramatic dialogue, we also find abundant use of Chinese idioms, which increase the difficulty for translators of the play. Example 1.3 reveals two different strategies of translating a Chinese idiom in the ST. In TT1, the allusion to the eight immortals in Chinese culture is "literally" translated; while in TT2, it is translated in a "free" way and is regarded as more suitable to be performed (cf. Yang 2016).

Example 1.3 (adapted from Lao 1999: 40–41, 2004: 40–41)

ST: 咱们 就 八 仙 过 海，各 显 其 能 吧！

PY: zán men jiù bā xiān guò hǎi, gè xiǎn qí néng ba

IG: we VADV eight immortal cross sea, each show his strength MOD

BT: We are like the eight immortals crossing the sea and each revealing his power!

TT1: Like the Eight Immortals crossing the sea, we each have our own strengths, eh?

TT2: Let's both try our best, and see what happens.

Dramatic monologue, different from the dialogues frequently found in drama, is "a speech of extended length and internal coherence, delivered by a single speaker, that does not include another's response" (Vince 2010: 402). A monologue can be addressed to the audience, the speaker himself or herself, another character, or even an object. In *Teahouse*, all dramatic monologues are addressed to the audience by a character called Shǎ Yáng, who is a beggar that earns a living by chanting rhythmic storytelling, translated as Oddball Young and Silly Young in TT1 and TT2 respectively.[1] The character was created by Lao She based on suggestions from directors and actors at Beijing People's Art Theater, with the aim of introducing the background of the eras and the other characters to the audience, as well as providing more time for actors to change their makeup between the two acts (Jiao 2007; Zhang 2008). Acting as the very first actor who approaches the audience in this play, Silly Young chants his lines by beating his clapper made of ox bone before the curtain rises. Then, after the curtain rises, he steps into the teahouse, interacts with the other characters, and asks for money from the manager of the teahouse. In this way, he also helps connect the plot in the three acts of the play.

According to Tam (2004: xxxviii), the dramatic monologue includes various "narrative elements of a Brechtian epic drama." Through the voice of Silly Young, Lao She not only describes the historical background to fill in the structural gaps between the three acts but also comments on the great changes in the society from the point of view of a beggar – one from a low social stratum. For instance, at the beginning of Act Three, Silly Young tells about the goings-on both in China and within the teahouse under the Japanese domination:

The Japs held old Beijing for eight long years,
Those were the days of blood and tears.
For those who survived, life was hell on earth,
The Eighth Route Army's victories, the only source of mirth.

> Hoping against hope such days would soon be past,
> Till the day came when the war was won at last.
> Then to old Beijing came the KMT!
> As cruel a tyrant as the Japs could ever be.
> Poor old Wang, disillusioned through and through,
> Keeping alive is all that he can do.
> His teahouse collapsing before his eyes,
> Won't perk up, no matter what he tries.
> What in the heavens above or the earth below,
> Can stop the officials from having all the dough?
> (Lao 1999: 239–241)

Stage direction, also called didascalia, refers to the "notes added to the script of a play to convey information about its performance not already explicit in the dialogue" (Hartnoll & Found 1996: 518). In *Teahouse*, all texts not spoken by actors belong to this category, and the playwright uses them to introduce the functions of the teahouse as well as instruct directors and actors of the play. At the beginning of Act One, we find a description of the cultural functions of Yutai Teahouse, which foreshadows the play's plot:

> Tea was served as well as simple snacks and quick meals. Bird fanciers, after having spent what they considered sufficient time strolling about with their caged orioles and thrushes, used to come here every day to rest, sip tea and demonstrate the singing virtuosity of their birds. The teahouse was also a meeting place for all sorts of discussions and transactions, and a haven for go-betweens and pimps.
> (Lao 1999: 3)

Also, by comparing the descriptions of the stage set, readers are acquainted with the historical background. In Act One, the teahouse is decorated in the following manner:

> Immediately inside the entrance we see the counter and the brick stove. . . . The building is extremely large and high, with rectangular tables, square tables, benches and stools for the customers. Through the window an inner courtyard can be seen, where there is a matted canopy for shade and seats for customers. There are devices for hanging up bird-cages, both in the teahouse and in the courtyard. Paper slips, with "Do not discuss affairs of state" written on them, are pasted all over the place.
> (Lao 1999: 5–7)

In the stage direction of Act Two, however, one finds both similarities and differences in the stage set. Despite the changes of layout in the teahouse, the notice, i.e. "Do not discuss affairs of state" is kept and even highlighted:

> The stove has been moved to the back, for preparing meals for the lodgers. The teahouse has undergone a great improvement too. The tables are now

smaller, with pale green table-cloths and wicker chairs. The huge painting of "the intoxicated eight immortals" on the wall and the shrine of the god of wealth have disappeared. In their place are posters of fashionably dressed beauty-queens – advertisements for foreign cigarette manufacturers. The "Do not discuss affairs of state" slips, however, have survived, written in an even larger script.

(Lao 1999: 59–61)

1.3 Analytical framework and data size

As a highly valued text, *Teahouse* has been examined from various perspectives, including functional equivalence, cooperative principle, skopos, etc., but has seldom been investigated through the lens of SFL (cf. Ren 2008). By using SFL, we reveal the various meaning-making resources in the texts analyzed and then compare the analysis made in the ST and the two TTs. However, we cannot analyze the texts in terms of all systems of language and have to be selective in building the analytical framework.

Before developing a suitable framework, we conducted a pilot study to have an overview of the linguistic features in the play using 50 clauses selected from each type of text, both in the ST and the TTs. Choices made by Lao She in the ST and the two translators in the TTs were analyzed in terms of the major systems, including THEME,[2] MOOD, MODALITY, POLARITY, TRANSITIVITY, TAXIS, and LOGICO-SEMANTIC TYPE. As shown in Example 1.4 (see Table 1.1), we analyzed the clause from the ST from the textual, interpersonal, and experiential perspectives. The analyses were then compared with those done in the TTs to ascertain the systems in which the differences between the ST and the TTs were most likely to be observed.

Moreover, analyses were made in the logical systems of TAXIS and LOGICO-SEMANTIC TYPE in the pilot study. Example 1.5 (see Table 1.2) illustrates how the

Table 1.1 Example 1.4

ST	唐先生,	你	外边	蹓蹓	吧 !	
PY	táng xiān sheng	nǐ	wài biān	liù liù	ba	
IG	Mr. Tang	you	outside	walk	MOD	
textual analysis	Theme		Rheme			interpersonal Theme: 唐先生 topical Theme: 你
interpersonal analysis	Vocative	Subject	Adjunct	Predicator		MOOD TYPE: imperative: jussive POLARITY: positive MODALITY: –
experiential analysis		Actor	Place	Process		PROCESS TYPE: material

Source: Adapted from Lao (2004: 15)

Table 1.2 Example 1.5

tactic structure	TT2
1	But I'd better stop
+2	and hold myself in check,
×3	Talking too freely will surely risk my neck!

Source: Adapted from Lao (1999: 233)

tactic structures between the three clauses were identified. In terms of taxis, the choice of parataxis was selected. In terms of logico-semantic type, the choice between the first two clauses was extension (+) and that between the last two clauses was enhancement (×). By the same token, choices made in the ST and the two TTs were compared using these parameters.

Based on the pilot study, the following observations were made:

1   For dramatic dialogue, the choices between the ST and the TTs vary especially from the interpersonal perspective in the system of MOOD.
2   For dramatic monologue, we find differences from the textual perspective in the system of THEME. Choices made in other systems do not vary to such a large extent.
3   For stage direction, similarities are found in the choices made in the systems of THEME, MOOD, MODALITY, POLARITY, and TRANSITIVITY between the ST and the TTs, while differences are observed in the SYSTEMS OF TAXIS and LOGICO-SEMANTIC TYPE.

Therefore, in the analytical framework (see Figure 1.7), we include the lexico-grammatical systems that tend to reveal more differences between the ST and the TTs. As a result, the analysis of dramatic dialogue will focus on the systems of MOOD, with considerations of the semantic system of SPEECH FUNCTION (see Chapter 2). The analysis of dramatic monologue will be based on the choices in the system of THEME (see Chapter 3). The analysis of stage direction will report on the analysis in the systems of TAXIS and LOGICO-SEMANTIC TYPE (see Chapter 4). Taken together, these selected systemic analyses will offer a revealing account of how the discourse of *Teahouse* is organized to effectively function in its context of situation and context of culture.

After the lexicogrammatical analysis, we will explore the contextual stratum by considering the three contextual parameters, i.e. field, tenor, and mode, in the comparison of the differences between the ST, TT1, and TT2. On the one hand, the three contextual parameters are significant in that they are capable of providing proofs for the interpretation of the differences identified in the lexicogrammatical analysis. On the other hand, variations in context are likely to influence the translators' choices, thus leading to the differences found in the lexicogrammatical analysis. In relation to lexicogrammar and context, the

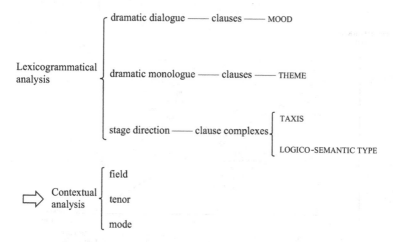

Figure 1.7 Analytical framework

features of mood revealed in the lexicogrammatical analysis will reflect the tenor – the interpersonal relations in the discourse. The analysis of Theme will be related to the mode of the discourse, informing us how the discourse is organized and planned. The analysis of taxis and logico-semantic type will help us identify the field of discourse and how spoken and written mode in the text is constructed.

The similarities and differences between the ST, TT1, and TT2 are expected to be identified based on the analysis. The analytical framework draws on various dimensions in the environments of translation (Matthiessen 2001). From the perspective of stratification, the analytical framework takes three strata into consideration, i.e. lexicogrammar, semantics, and context. Regarding metafunction, three are involved in the framework – interpersonal, textual, and logical. In terms of rank, translation is examined by measuring the translation equivalence and shift on the clause rank. Also, along the cline of instantiation, the analysis proceeds from the instance pole of the cline and moves to the subsystem or the system pole.

After the analysis and comparison, some reasons that lead to the different choices in the ST, TT1, and TT2 will be identified, which can be categorized as (i) systemic, i.e. due to the systemic contrast between Chinese and English; (ii) registerial, i.e. choices are made in consideration of register; (iii) instantiated, i.e. choices are largely personal, based on the translator's own judgment or related to the translators' habitus (see Hansen & Hansen-Schirra 2012 for a summary of the three types of reasons).

After constructing the analytical framework, we need to determine the data size in the analysis. As shown in Figure 1.8, studies can be located on the cline between

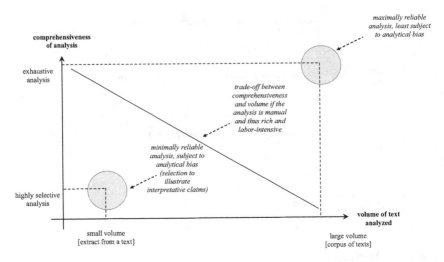

Figure 1.8 Relationship between comprehensiveness of analysis and volume of text analyzed

Source: Adapted from Matthiessen (2014a: 189)

minimally reliable analysis and maximally reliable analysis, on which Matthiessen (2014a: 188) has made the following observation:

> Minimally reliable analysis simply means that very few systems have been considered in the analysis, and the analysis has been applied to a very small volume of text, such as an extract from a single text. Maximally reliable analysis means that the analysis involves as wide a range of systems as possible, and that it has been applied to a very large volume of text.

To make our study more reliable, trade-offs have to be made between comprehensiveness of analysis and volume of text involved. In the analytical framework, we try to make our analysis comprehensive, which involves a selective number of systems instead of being exhaustive. Also, we try to include a relatively large volume of text, despite the fact that the analysis will be manual and labor intensive. Thus, the data to be analyzed are selected in the following way: (i) the analysis of dramatic dialogue in Chapter 2 will involve the first act in the ST, TT1, and TT2; (ii) the analysis of dramatic monologue in Chapter 3 will be based on the complete ST and the two TTs; (iii) the analysis of stage direction in Chapter 4 will be carried out on the beginning paragraphs in the three acts, which serve the introductory purposes by providing information about the stage setting and the major characters. We exclude the latter parts of stage direction that intersect with the dramatic dialogue to give directions to actors and abound

Table 1.3 Number of clauses in the data

	ST	TT1	TT2
dramatic dialogue	571	586	567
dramatic monologue	161	138	140
stage direction	125	110	109

with non-Finite clauses in the TTs such as "coming over" (Lao 1999: 111) and "seeing Master Chang" (Lao 1999: 89). Table 1.3 tabulates the number of clauses selected for the analysis.

Notes

1 Since the Ming Dynasty but before 1949, these professional beggars did not beg for food, but instead asked for money. The rhythmic storytelling that the beggars chant is called "数来宝" (shǔ lái bǎo) or "快板" (kuài bǎn) in Chinese, characterized by simple and humorous words, sometimes vulgar and obscene, and composed in a rhymed and rhythmic pattern. The instrument they used can be either bamboo sticks or two pieces of ox bones decorated with little bells. The beggars might not have had a fixed place for performance, so they made their rounds from shop to shop (cf. Lian 2012; Shih 2012).

2 We follow Halliday and Matthiessen's (2014) convention of technical terms in SFL. For instance, MOOD is used to refer to the name of the grammatical system of the speech function, and MOOD is the element in the interpersonal structure of the English clause.

2 Reenacting interpersonal meaning in dramatic dialogue

This chapter reports on the interpersonal analysis of mood in the dramatic dialogue of *Teahouse* and its two English translations. Section 2.1 provides a brief introduction to the system of MOOD. Section 2.2 discusses the findings of the mood analysis, pointing out the choices made in the ST and the TTs, and relating the choices of mood to the characterization of the play. Section 2.3 discusses the mood shifts found, introduces the various categories of mood shifts, and explains the reasons for such shifts.

2.1 A description of mood in systemic functional terms

Mood, also referred to as mood type, is the primary interpersonal system of the clause. Modeled on the interpersonal metafunction, mood deals with the interpersonal organization of the clause as a move in an exchange. It is the realization of the semantic system of SPEECH FUNCTION in lexicogrammar, and it incorporates various subsystems, such as polarity, freedom, mood assessment, comment, subject person, finiteness, and modality type. According to the description of English lexicogrammar (see Matthiessen 1995a; Halliday & Matthiessen 2014), all major clauses make a selection in the system of MOOD, realizing the speech functions of the moves that they enact. As shown in Figure 2.1, a major clause can be indicative or imperative. If it is indicative, it can be either declarative or interrogative. If it is interrogative, it can be further refined into yes/no interrogative and wh-interrogative.

In the system of MOOD, speakers, writers, and their addressees are involved in interactive events. When a speaker adopts a certain speech role, s/he simultaneously assigns a complementary role to the listener. The two basic types of speech role in the system of ORIENTATION include giving and demanding (see Table 2.1). There is another fundamental distinction of the interaction, i.e. the nature of the commodity being exchanged – whether it is goods and services or information. When orientation is combined with the commodity exchanged, we have four basic speech functions, namely "offer," "statement," "command," and "question."

Within the interpersonal structure of the clause in English, the Mood element – composed of Subject, Finite, and modal Adjunct – makes a key contribution. "The Subject is the element in terms of which the clause can be negotiated," while "the Finite makes a clause negotiable by coding it as positive or negative in polarity

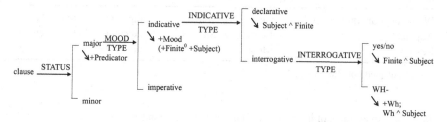

Figure 2.1 The system network of MOOD in English

Source: Adapted from Halliday & Matthiessen (2014: 24)

Table 2.1 Four types of exchanges and the speech functions

role in exchange	Commodity exchanged	
	(a) goods and services	*(b) information*
(i) giving	"offer" I'll give you a cup of tea?	"statement" Life will never be easy.
(ii) demanding	"command" Have a look at this!	"question" How much does it cost?

Source: from Halliday & Matthiessen (2014: 136)

and by grounding it, either in terms of time (it is/it isn't; it was/it wasn't; it will/it won't) or in terms of modality (it may/it will/it must, etc.)" (Martin, Matthiessen & Painter 2010: 61). At the same time, there is modal Adjunct, which adds "meaning related to the mood element: polarity and modality (e.g. perhaps, probably, certainly), temporality (e.g. already, soon, yet) and intensity (e.g. degree: hardly, quite, almost, totally, utterly; counter-expectancy: even, actually, just, simply, merely, only)" (ibid.). The syntagmatic order of Subject and Finite determines the mood types in English. For instance, when Subject is followed by Finite, the mood type is declarative; when Finite precedes Subject, the mood type is yes/no interrogative. In addition to Subject and Finite, there are other elements excluded in the Mood structure, namely Residue, which is made up of Predicator, Complement, and Adjunct, with the Predicator being the non-Finite part of the verbal group, the Complement being a nominal group, and the Adjunct being the adverbial group or prepositional phrase (see Table 2.2 for example).

According to the description of Mandarin Chinese (e.g. Halliday & McDonald 2004; Li 2007), the basic choices in the system of MOOD are similar to those in English. However, as the concept of finiteness does not exist in Chinese, mood type cannot be differentiated according to the syntagmatic order of Subject and Finite. Table 2.3 illustrates an analysis of a clause in Chinese. The mood type of the clause is polar interrogative of the biassed subtype and is realized by the modal particle "吧" (PY: ba; IG: MOD) found at the end of the clause and the question mark.

Table 2.2 An example of interpersonal analysis in a clause in English

Where in your whole village	can	you	scrape up	ten taels?
Adjunct	Finite	Subject	Predicator	Complement
Resi-	Mood		-due	

Source: Adapted from Lao (1999: 23)

Table 2.3 An example of interpersonal analysis in a clause in Chinese

你	听说过	庞总管	吧？
nǐ	tīng shuō guò	páng zǒng guǎn	ba
you	hear of	Eunuch Pang	MOD
Subject	Predicator	Complement	

Source: Adapted from Lao (1999: 20)

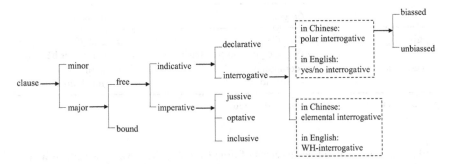

Figure 2.2 Differences in the system of MOOD between English and Mandarin

Also, different from English, the Subject in a major clause in Chinese has the potential to be omitted. Systemically, the two languages contrast with each other in their choices of interrogative (see Figure 2.2): in English, an interrogative can be either yes/no or wh- interrogative, while in Chinese, the choices include polar and elemental. We also note that despite similar paradigmatic choices of mood in the two languages, the syntagmatic realizations of these choices are different. More examples of such differences will be summarized in Section 2.4.

2.2 Analysis of mood in dramatic dialogue

Dramatic dialogue is composed of dialogic exchanges. Therefore, it is suitable to apply the grammar of interaction to investigate the interpersonal choices made by the two translators. We first report on the quantitative findings of mood analysis and then relate the different kinds of mood types with the major characters in the play, such as Wang Lifa, Pock-Mark Liu, Master Chang, and Qin Zhongyi. In addition, we provide an analysis of moodtags found in the data.

Table 2.4 Distribution of mood in the analysis of dramatic dialogue

Mood type			ST	TT1	TT2
indicative	interrogative	declarative	304	293	286
		polar in the ST yes/no in the TT	44	16	17
		elemental in the ST wh- in the TT	35	39	42
	imperative		95	69	82
	bound		38	98	73
	minor		55	71	66
	Total		572	586	566

2.2.1 A quantitative profile of mood distribution in dramatic dialogue[1]

After the lexicogrammatical analysis of mood choices, an overall distribution of mood in the data of dramatic dialogue has been presented in Table 2.4.

By comparing the distribution of mood in the ST and the two TTs, we find that in the TTs, there has been a decrease in most types of free clauses, i.e. declaratives, polar interrogatives, and imperatives, and an increase in bound and minor clauses. To interpret the quantitative differences (though the numbers are not significantly varied) and to find some patterns in translating the dramatic dialogue in *Teahouse*, we further relate the analysis of mood to the different characters in the play, as the analysis of mood can help us understand the creation and recreation of the characters (cf. Yu & Wu 2016).

Despite the different strategies adopted by the two translators, a similar frequency of mood distribution is observed between the ST and the TTs. The general tendency is that more clauses are found in the ST, while in the TTs, especially in TT2, a smaller number of clauses are identified. Example 2.1 shows how two clauses in the ST are translated as one clause in both TTs, with the second clause in the ST being downranked to a "narrower" environment in terms of rank, suggesting the translators' preference to move in this direction (Matthiessen 2001). In other words, the second clause in the ST is translated as "not mine" – a nominal group in the two TTs.

Example 2.1 (adapted from Lao 1999: 20–21, 2004: 22–23)

ST: 那 是 你们 乡下 的 事, (mood type: declarative)
PY: nà shì nǐ men xiāng xià de shì
IG: that be your countryside SUB problem
BT: That's your problem in the countryside,
我 管 不 着。(mood type: declarative)
PY: wǒ guǎn bù zháo
IG: I care NEG VADV
BT: I don't care.
TT1: That's you peasants' problem, not mine. (mood type: declarative)
TT2: That's your problem, not mine! (mood type: declarative)

In addition, the frequencies of bound clauses in the two TTs increase, suggesting the use of different strategies by the two translators in terms of clause complexing, compared to the choices in the ST. As shown in Example 2.2, the second clause in the ST, a declarative, is translated as a bound clause in both TTs. Such strategies in translation indicate the translators' different choices in combining two clauses into one clause complex. In the ST, the logico-semantic relation between the two clauses is elaboration, represented as $1 = 2$. Clauses of equal status are used, with the second clause elaborating the "good deeds" mentioned in the first clause. Comparatively, in the two TTs, the logico-semantic relations are rendered as those of enhancement, represented as $\alpha \times \beta$. The relations between the two clauses are unequal, with the second clauses being bound ones and enhancing relations being used to link the two clauses.

Example 2.2 (adapted from Lao 1999: 36–37, 2004: 36–37)

ST: 常四爷，您 是 积德行好，(mood type: declarative)
PY: cháng sì yé, nín shì jī dé xíng hǎo
IG: Master Chang you (HON) EMPH do good deeds
BT: Master Chang, you do good deeds,
赏给 她们 面 吃！(mood type: declarative)
PY: shǎng gěi tā men miàn chī
IG: grant them noodle eat
BT: grant them noodles to eat.
TT1: Fourth Elder Chang, it's very good of you (mood type: declarative) to buy them noodles. (mood type: bound)
TT2: Master Chang, you're really softhearted (mood type: declarative) giving them noodles! (mood type: bound)

In general, mood types in the ST are often maintained in the TTs. Example 2.3 shows how a declarative in the ST is translated or reenacted equivalently as declaratives in both TTs. We also note that equivalence is not only found in the lexicogrammatical system of MOOD but also in the semantic system of SPEECH FUNCTION. In this extract, Pock-Mark Liu is persuading Kang Liu to sell his daughter to Eunuch Pang by boasting about the wealth of Eunuch Pang. The speech function of the clause in the ST is "statement," which remains unchanged in the TTs.

Example 2.3 (adapted from Lao 1999: 20–21, 2004: 24–25)

ST: 连 家 里 打 醋 的 瓶子 都 是 玛瑙 做 的! (mood type: declarative; speech function: statement)
PY: lián jiā lǐ dǎ cù de píng zi dōu shì mǎ nǎo zuò de
IG: even home in contain vinegar SUB bottle all be agate make SUB
BT: Even the vinegar bottle in his home is made of agate!
TT1: Even his vinegar bottles are made of agate. (mood type: declarative; speech function: statement)
TT2: Even the vinegar bottle in his house is made of agate! (mood type: declarative; speech function: statement)

Though similar in proportion, the mood choices in the ST and the TTs are not always equivalent. For instance, we find a reduction in the frequencies of declarative, yes/no interrogative, imperative: jussive, and imperative: optative, and increases in the occurrences of wh- interrogative and bound clauses. These mood shifts are not made randomly but are closely related to the translators' recreation of the characters. For instance, to enhance the cruelty of Pock-Mark Liu, his declaratives addressed to Kang Liu are often translated as wh- interrogatives or imperatives, which convey a threatening tone to the addressee (see Section 2.2.2). In addition, such shifts are seen in both TT1 and TT2, but with a higher frequency in TT2, as the translator of TT2 adopts a freer way of translation and focuses on performability.

Teahouse is famous for its vivid depiction of the characters (cf. Cao 2007; Ying 1999, 2007). The translator of TT2, Ying Ruocheng, also thinks highly of Lao She's distinctive style of characterization. In his view, even "merely one line in the play is capable of depicting one character" (Ying 1999: 6, our translation; cf. Ying & Conceison 2009). As shown in Table 2.5, 12 characters in Act One of *Teahouse* are selected for the analysis. Some characters, who only have a few lines or whose contributions are minor clauses (e.g. the anonymous customers in the teahouse, the little girl sold by her mother, and Kang Shunz), are ignored here. From Section 2.2.2 to 2.2.12, we will discuss the mood choices in the ST and the TTs in relation to the characterization of the play.

2.2.2 Mood analysis of Pock-Mark Liu's lines

Pock-Mark Liu, first played by the translator of the TT2 (Ying Ruocheng) on stage, is a professional human trafficker and an antagonist of the play. An analysis of the mood type of the ST shows that he contributes the highest number of interrogatives and a relatively high number of imperatives among all characters in Act One. Most interrogatives and imperatives are addressed to Kang Liu – the peasant who sells his daughter to Pock-Mark Liu. Some imperatives are also addressed to Master Song to invite him to purchase a tiny watch. Semantically, the mood types of interrogatives and imperatives realize the speech functions of "question" and "command." However, while speaking to a powerful person like Eunuch Pang, a high-ranking official and the buyer of Kang Liu's daughter, only declaratives are found in Pock-Mark Liu's free clauses in the ST.

In the TTs, when Pock-Mark Liu talks to Kang Liu, who has a low social status, the interrogatives are often translated as declaratives by both translators to add more certainty to Pock-Mark Liu's assertions. Examples 2.4 and 2.5 illustrate how interrogatives are translated as declaratives in TT2. In Example 2.4, a biassed subtype of interrogative is translated as a declarative in TT2, resulting in a shift of mood type. Such a shift makes Pock-Mark Liu's remark more persuasive in compelling Kang Liu to sell his daughter. On hearing this, Kang Liu is forced to believe that his daughter is lucky to marry a eunuch who is powerful and rich. However, in TT1, equivalence is maintained in terms of mood but with respect to delicacy, as there are neither biassed nor unbiassed subtypes of interrogatives in English. Thus, the translation in English cannot be as delicate as the ST.

Table 2.5 Main characters and the distribution of mood in the analysis of dramatic dialogue

Character	Text	Mood type						
		declarative	interrogative		imperative	bound	minor	Total
			polar yes/no	elemental wh-				
刘麻子 Pock-Mark Liu	ST	66 (60.6%)	10 (9.2%)	4 (3.7%)	16 (15%)	10 (9.2%)	3 (2.8%)	109
	TT1	55 (52.9%)	4 (3.8%)	7 (6.7%)	14 (13.5%)	17 (16.8%)	6 (5.8%)	104
	TT2	55 (56.1%)	3 (3.1%)	7 (7.1%)	15 (15.3%)	17 (18.4%)	3 (3.1%)	98
王利发 Wang Lifa	ST	54 (50.9%)	6 (5.7%)	4 (3.8%)	28 (26.4%)	8 (7.5%)	6 (5.7%)	106
	TT1	48 (45.7%)	3 (2.9%)	8 (7.6%)	17 (16.2%)	23 (21.9%)	6 (5.7%)	105
	TT2	51 (50.5%)	3 (3%)	8 (7.9%)	18 (17.8%)	12 (11.9%)	9 (8.9%)	101
常四爷 Master Chang	ST	30 (55.6%)	2 (3.7%)	6 (11.1%)	8 (14.8%)	4 (7.4%)	4 (7.4%)	54
	TT1	26 (48.1%)	1 (1.9%)	7 (13%)	4 (7.4%)	13 (24.1%)	3 (5.6%)	54
	TT2	23 (41.8%)	1 (3.6%)	9 (16.4%)	10 (18.2%)	9 (16.1%)	3 (5.5%)	55
秦仲义 Qin Zhongyi	ST	33 (62.3%)	2 (3.8%)	1 (1.9%)	9 (17%)	3 (5.7%)	5 (9.4%)	53
	TT1	35 (58.3%)	1 (1.7%)	1 (1.7%)	6 (10%)	10 (16.7%)	7 (11.7%)	60
	TT2	29 (52.7%)	2 (3.6%)	1 (1.8%)	6 (10.9%)	9 (16.4%)	8 (14.5%)	55
康六 Kang Liu	ST	14 (38.9%)	3 (8.3%)	7 (19.4%)	2 (5.6%)	1 (2.8%)	9 (25%)	36
	TT1	13 (31.7%)	3 (7.3%)	6 (14.6%)	1 (2.4%)	6 (14.6%)	12 (29.3%)	41
	TT2	15 (41.7%)	1 (2.8%)	7 (19.4%)	2 (5.6%)	3 (8.3%)	8 (22.2%)	36
松二爷 Master Song	ST	12 (34.3%)	3 (8.6%)	4 (11.4%)	11 (31.4%)	0	5 (14.3%)	35
	TT1	15 (42.9%)	0	3 (8.6%)	10 (28.6%)	3 (8.6%)	4 (11.4%)	35
	TT2	15 (40.5%)	3 (8.1%)	4 (10.8%)	9 (24.3%)	1 (2.7%)	5 (13.5%)	37
庞太监 Eunuch Pang	ST	18 (56.3%)	5 (15.6%)	1 (3.1%)	4 (12.5%)	1 (3.1%)	3 (9.4%)	32
	TT1	18 (60%)	1 (3.3%)	1 (3.3%)	1 (3.3%)	5 (16.7%)	4 (13.3%)	30
	TT2	16 (45.7%)	1 (2.9%)	2 (5.7%)	3 (8.6%)	5 (14.3%)	8 (22.9%)	35

唐铁嘴 Tang the Oracle	ST	14 (70%)	0	0	3 (15%)	1 (5%)	2 (10%)	20
	TT1	11 (57.9%)	0	0	4 (21.1%)	2 (10.5%)	2 (10.5%)	19
	TT2	10 (62.5%)	0	1 (6.3%)	2 (12.5%)	1 (6.3%)	2 (12.5%)	16
二德子 Erdez	ST	9 (52.9%)	2 (11.8%)	2 (11.8%)	2 (11.8%)	1 (5.9%)	1 (5.9%)	17
	TT1	12 (60%)	0	1 (5%)	1 (5%)	2 (10%)	4 (20%)	20
	TT2	10 (58.8%)	0	1 (5.9%)	2 (11.8%)	1 (5.9%)	3 (17.6%)	17
宋恩子 Song Enz	ST	8 (50%)	2 (12.5%)	0	4 (25%)	2 (12.5%)	0	16
	TT1	11 (68.8%)	1 (6.3%)	0	1 (6.3%)	1 (6.3%)	2 (12.5%)	16
	TT2	10 (58.8%)	0	0	3 (17.6%)	2 (11.8%)	2 (11.8%)	17
李三 Li San	ST	5 (41.7%)	0	1 (8.3%)	5 (41.7%)	0	1 (8.3%)	12
	TT1	10 (71.4%)	0	0	2 (14.3%)	0	2 (14.3%)	14
	TT2	8 (61.5%)	0	0	2 (15.4%)	2 (15.4%)	1 (7.7%)	13
吴祥子 Wu Xiangz	ST	2 (28.6%)	3 (42.9%)	0	1 (14.3%)	1 (14.3%)	0	7
	TT1	4 (57.1%)	0	0	1 (14.3%)	2 (28.6%)	0	7
	TT2	3 (50%)	1 (16.7%)	0	1 (16.7%)	1 (16.7%)	0	6

Example 2.4 (adapted from Lao 1999: 20–21, 2004: 24–25)

ST: 那 不 是 你 女儿 的 命 好 吗？(mood type: interrogative: polar: biassed)
PY: nà bú shì nǐ nǚ er de mìng hǎo ma
IG: that NEG be your daughter SUB fate good MOD
BT: Doesn't your daughter have good fate?
TT1: So then, isn't your daughter lucky? (mood type: interrogative: yes/no)
TT2: That's why your daughter's a lucky girl! (mood type: declarative)

Similarly, in Example 2.5, the interrogative in the ST is translated as declaratives
in both TTs, resulting in shifts in mood type. We also find the use of modality in
the two TTs, i.e. "surely" in TT1 and "must" in TT2, which both modulate probability. Moreover, such shifts in mood type represent changes from indirectness to
directness, from orientation toward addressees to orientation toward content, and
from implicitness to explicitness. These patterns coincide with House's (1998)
dimensions of cross-cultural differences in translation (see Blum-Kulka & House
1989; House 1996; Figure 2.3). Although the language pair in the present study is
different from the one in House (1998), some similar shifts from one end of the
cline to the other end are observed in the TTs.

Example 2.5 (adapted from Lao 1999: 20–21, 2004: 24–25)

ST: 你 也 听说过 庞总管 吧？(mood type: interrogative: polar: biassed)
PY: nǐ yě tīng shuō guò páng zǒng guǎn ba
IG: you also hear of Eunuch Pang MOD
BT: Have you also heard of Eunuch Pang?
TT1: Surely you've heard of him. (mood type: declarative)
TT2: Even you must have heard of him. (mood type: declarative)

For the declaratives addressed to Kang Liu, we find that they tend to be translated
as wh- interrogatives or imperatives. As a cruel individual, Pock-Mark Liu threatens Kang Liu and urges him to quickly make up his mind to sell his daughter.
While translating, the two translators often choose interrogatives and imperatives,

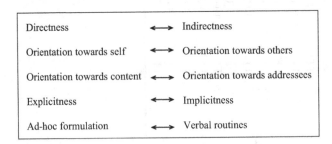

Figure 2.3 Dimensions of cross-cultural difference

Source: Adapted from House (1998: 62)

which further reinforce the wickedness of Pock-Mark Liu. In Example 2.6, we observe a mood shift when the two declaratives in the ST are translated as the jussive subtype of imperative in both TTs. A dynamic equivalent translation, rather than a literal translation about nodding one's head, helps the translators to portray the wickedness of the human trafficker.

Example 2.6 (adapted from Lao 1999: 20–21, 2004: 24–25)

ST: 摇 头 不 算 (mood type: declarative)
PY: yáo tóu bú suàn
IG: shake head NEG count
BT: Shaking head does not count,
点 头 算。(mood type: declarative)
PY: diǎn tóu suàn
IG: nod head count
BT: nodding head counts.
TT1: Well, make up your mind (mood type: imperative: jussive)
TT2: Well, make up your mind, yes or no. (mood type: imperative: jussive)

Similar mood shifts are more frequent in TT2. As shown in Examples 2.7 and 2.8, the translator of TT2 chooses to change the declarative mood in the ST, while the translator of TT1 chooses to maintain the equivalence of the declarative mood. In Example 2.7, the declarative in the ST is changed to the wh- subcategory of interrogative in TT2, leading to the change of speech function from "statement" to "question." In TT1, while the declarative is translated equivalently in TT1, a mood tag is added, which functions similarly as the interrogative in TT2 that demands an answer from Kang Liu – the addressee. Example 2.8 illustrates how a declarative is translated as an imperative in TT2, thereby making Pock-Mark Liu's language more forceful and achieving the aim of threatening Kang Liu to accept his fate and to make the deal.

Example 2.7 (adapted from Lao 1999: 20–21, 2004: 24–25)

ST: [ø:你] 也 对不起 女儿! (mood type: declarative)
PY: nǐ yě duì bù qǐ nǚ er
IG: you also sorry for daughter
BT: You are also sorry for your daughter!
TT1: You won't be able to face her again, will you? (mood type: declarative: tagged: reversed polarity)
TT2: How can you face her anyway? (mood type: interrogative: wh-)

Example 2.8 (adapted from Lao 1999: 20–21, 2004: 24–25)

ST: 你 糊涂! (mood type: declarative)
PY: nǐ hú tu
IG: you foolish

BT: You are foolish!
TT1: You are a fool. (mood type: declarative)
TT2: Don't be a fool! (mood type: imperative: jussive)

However, when translating Pock-Mark Liu's lines addressed to Master Song and Master Chang, two regular Manchurian customers as well as Liu's potential customers, different strategies of selecting the mood types are adopted by the translators. In Examples 2.9, 2.10, and 2.11, imperatives of the jussive subtype are used in the ST, which demand Master Song and Master Chang to try the tea, to keep the watch, or to pay later. In the TTs, especially in TT2, such imperatives tend to be translated as declaratives, with modulated uses of modality often added, such as "must" in Example 2.9, "had better" and "ought to" in Example 2.10, and "can" in Example 2.11. For the translators, it is natural to recreate the image of Pock-Mark Liu in this way – moving from directness to indirectness and from explicitness to implicitness, which is opposite to the strategy used in translating Pock-Mark Liu's lines to Kang Liu, because the two Manchurian customers have a much higher status than Kang Liu's, as Kang is merely a poor peasant.

Example 2.9 (adapted from Lao 1999: 18–19, 2004: 22–23)

ST: 您 试试 这个! (mood type: imperative: jussive)
PY: nín shì shì zhèi ge
IG: you (HON) try this
BT: Try this!
TT1: Try this! (mood type: imperative: jussive)
TT2: You must try this. (mood type: declarative)

Example 2.10 (adapted from Lao 1999: 26–27, 2004: 28–29)

ST: 松二爷，留 下 这个 表 吧, (mood type: imperative: jussive)
PY: sōng èr yé, liú xià zhèi ge biǎo ba
IG: Master Song keep CV this watch MOD
BT: Master Song, keep this watch!
TT1: Second Elder Song, you'd better hang onto that watch. (mood type: declarative)
TT2: Master Song, you really ought to keep this watch. (mood type: declarative)

Example 2.11 (adapted from Lao 1999: 26–27, 2004: 28–29)

ST: [ø:您] 改 日 再 给 钱! (mood type: imperative: jussive)
PY: nín gǎi rì zài gěi qián
IG: you (HON) another day VADV pay money
BT: Pay me another day!
TT1: Pay me later. (mood type: imperative: jussive)
TT2: You can pay later. (mood type: declarative)

Another character that Pock-Mark Liu interacts with is Eunuch Pang, a prestigious official in the royal court and the buyer of Kang Liu's daughter. In the ST, all Pock-Mark Liu's free clauses addressed to Eunuch Pang are declaratives. Taking tenor into consideration, we find that Eunuch Pang's social status is much higher than that of Pock-Mark Liu. Thus, the speech functions of such moves are mostly "statement" and "offer," realized by declaratives in lexicogrammar, indicating Pock-Mark Liu's willingness to work for Eunuch Pang and emphasizing how hard-working he has been. The two translators have maintained the social status between the two characters and do not shift in this respect by translating the declaratives equivalently (see Example 2.12).

Example 2.12 (adapted from Lao 1999: 44–45, 2004: 42–43)

ST: 一丝一毫 不 能 马虎! (mood type: declarative)
PY: yì sī yì háo bù néng mǎ hu
IG: a tiny bit NEG can careless
BT: I cannot be careless to a tiny bit.
TT1: I haven't left a single thing to chance. (mood type: declarative)
TT2: I left no stone unturned. (mood type: declarative)

2.2.3 Mood analysis of Wang Lifa's lines

Wang Lifa, the manager of Yutai Teahouse, is the protagonist of the play. To manage a teahouse in the turbulent days, he tries to closely follow his father's principle of communication, i.e. "always be polite, always make obeisance, try to please everybody" (Lao 2004: 31), as written by Lao She in the lines of Wang Lifa. He is clever and tactful while serving different kinds of customers. In Act One of the play, he is still young and is therefore energetic, diligent, and talkative (see Yu 2007).

The mood analysis of the ST reveals that Wang Lifa adopts different linguistic strategies in dealing with different people. When interacting with people with a lower social status, such as Tang the Oracle and the little girl being sold by her mother, he uses various imperatives, which realize the speech function of "command." By using these imperatives, Wang Lifa orders these people to leave the teahouse. While speaking to Li San, who is the attendant in the teahouse, he mostly uses imperatives to order him to provide goods and services to other customers. When interacting with people of a higher social status, such as Qin Zhongyi, Eunuch Pang, Master Song, and Master Chang, Wang Lifa also uses some imperatives; however, the speech function of these imperatives is "offer," i.e. to provide goods and services, such as to give Qin Zhongyi or other customers a cup of tea. Many of such imperatives function as commands, i.e. to ask these people to take a seat. This explains why the highest number of imperatives are used by Wang Lifa in comparison with the other characters (see Table 2.5).

In the TTs, however, translation shifts involving the imperatives are frequently observed. These imperatives are sometimes translated as other mood types. They can be translated as wh- interrogatives, which reveal Wang Lifa's attempt to speak indirectly and implicitly instead of forcefully, actively, directly, and explicitly. Examples include the imperative that bids Tang the Oracle to leave the teahouse (see Example 2.13) and the imperative that invites Erdez to come to the inner courtyard (Example 2.14). In these two examples, mood shifts are involved when the imperatives in the ST are translated as interrogatives of the wh- subtype in both TTs.

Example 2.13 (adapted from Lao 1999: 8–9, 2004: 14–15)

ST: 唐先生, 你 外边 溜溜 吧! (mood type: imperative: jussive)

PY: táng xiān sheng, nǐ wài biān liù liu ba

IG: Mr. Tang you outside walk MOD

BT: Mr. Tang, take a walk outside!

TT1: Older Tang, why don't you take a walk, eh? (mood type: interrogative: wh-)

TT2: Mr Tang, why not take a walk somewhere else? (mood type: interrogative: wh-)

Example 2.14 (adapted from Lao 1999: 14–15, 2004: 18–19)

ST: 德爷, 您 后边 坐! (mood type: imperative: jussive)

PY: dé ye, nín hòu biān zuò

IG: Master Erdez you (HON) back sit

BT: Master Erdez, take a seat at the back.

TT1: Sir, why don't you join them in the inner courtyard? (mood type: interrogative: wh-)

TT2: Master Erdez, why not take a seat in the inner courtyard now? (mood type: interrogative: wh-)

The two translators adopt different strategies when translating Wang Lifa's imperatives addressed to Tang the Oracle. As shown in Example 2.15, the jussive subtype of imperative in the ST is translated as a declarative in TT1 and a wh- interrogative in TT2. The speech function then changes from "command" to "statement" and "question" respectively. Thus, Wang Lifa's strategy of refusing Tang the Oracle is marked out explicitly in the two TTs by either stating the futility of fortune-telling in TT1 or by directly questioning the significance of fortune-telling in TT2.

Example 2.15 (adapted from Lao 1999: 10–11, 2004: 14–15)

ST: [ø:你] 用 不 着 相面,   (mood type: imperative: jussive)

PY: nǐ yòng bù zháo xiàng miàn

IG: you need NEG VPART fortune telling

BT: You do not need to try fortunetelling.

TT1: Fortunetelling's useless. (mood type: declarative)

TT2: What's the point of fortune-telling? (mood type: interrogative: wh-)

Toward the end of Act One, Wang Lifa interacts with a little girl who is taken to the teahouse to be sold. An imperative is used to ask the girl to leave the teahouse (see Example 2.16). In TT1, this clause is translated equivalently as an imperative: jussive, whereas in TT2, it is changed to a declarative. Wang Lifa is not angry with the girl for staying in his teahouse. He wants her to leave because there is no way to help her in such a situation, as he said in a previous line, "there are many cases like this. . . . You can't help them all" (Lao 1999: 37). After seeing his regular customers – Master Chang and Master Song – arrested by the undercover agents, he is now feeling disillusioned and impotent (Yu 2007). The mood shift in TT2 and the added modulation "had better" both help to soften the tone.

Example 2.16 (adapted from Lao 1999: 34–35, 2004: 34–35)

ST: 出去 吧, (mood type: imperative: jussive)
PY: chū qu ba
IG: go out MOD
BT: Go out!
TT1: Out you go. (mood type: imperative: jussive)
TT2: You'd better go now. (mood type: declarative)

Furthermore, we find that the imperatives of all the three subtypes – jussive, optative, and suggestive/inclusive – addressed to Wang Lifa's regular customers or those with a higher status, such as Master Song, Master Chang, and the landlord (Qin Zhongyi), are frequently translated as declaratives or other mood types. Examples 2.17 and 2.18 display mood shifts of this kind, with modalities such as "can" being added.

Example 2.17 (adapted from Lao 1999: 18–19, 2004: 20–21)

ST: [ø: 咱们] 待会儿 再 算 吧! (mood type: imperative: suggestive)
PY: zán men dāi huì er zài suàn ba
IG: we later VADV settle MOD
BT: Let's settle this later.
TT1: We'll square up later. (mood type: declarative)
TT2: We can settle that later. (mood type: declarative)

Example 2.18 (adapted from Lao 1999: 36–37, 2004: 36–37)

ST: 您 别 那么 办 哪, 二爷! (mood type: imperative: jussive)
PY: nín bié nà me bàn na, èr yé
IG: you (HON) do NEG that do MOD, Second Elder
BT: Don't do that, Second Elder!
TT1: But you can't do that, Second Elder! (mood type: declarative)
TT2: But you can't do that, sir! (mood type: declarative)

2.2.4   Mood analysis of Master Chang's lines

Master Chang is an unyielding character who is brave enough to challenge Erdez, a hired thug that lords it over the others in the teahouse. He is patriotic in that he worries about the future of the Qing Empire and the money being spent on foreign goods. He is also kind-hearted in buying noodles for the poor girl and her mother (Zheng 1983, 2007; Pu 2007).

His personality is also reflected in the mood distribution in the ST. A large number of declaratives are addressed to Master Song while discussing state affairs, showing his concern about the empire. He addresses most imperatives to Erdez, Li San, and the two secret agents. In this way, he challenges Erdez over Erdez's impotence in fighting with the foreigners, he orders the noodles for the poor girl by addressing Li San, and he refuses the two secret agents' order to chain him during his arrest. As for the interrogatives, in terms of both the polar and the elemental subtypes, they are mostly either used to question Erdez before starting their fight or to ask the two secret agents about the law case he is involved in.

In the TTs, an imperative addressed to Master Song has been translated as a declarative and interrogative: yes/no in TT1 and TT2 respectively, for the sake of interacting with the addressee in an indirect way and showing mutual respect between the two friends (see Example 2.19). Realizations of modality are also found, including "should" in TT1 and "won't" in TT2.

Example 2.19 (adapted from Lao 1999: 12–13, 2004: 16–17)

ST: 您 喝 这个! (mood type: imperative: jussive)
PY: nín hē zhèi ge
IG: you (HON) drink this
BT: You drink this.
TT1: You should really try this. (mood type: declarative)
TT2: Won't you have some of this? (mood type: interrogative: yes/no)

For the clauses addressed to Erdez, different choices are made to translate the interrogatives and imperatives. For example, an interrogative: polar is translated as an interrogative: wh- to question Erdez for starting a fight (Example 2.20). In another example (Example 2.21), an interrogative: wh- is translated as a declarative in TT1 to syntagmatically maintain the equivalence of word order in the ST, with a question mark being added to indicate the speech function of "question." In addition, in Example 2.22, an imperative is translated as an interrogative: wh- in TT1 to infuriate Erdez and to reveal Erdez's impotence in fighting with the real enemies of the empire.

Example 2.20 (adapted from Lao 1999: 12–13, 2004: 16–17)

ST: 你 问 我 哪? (mood type: polar: biassed)
PY: nǐ wèn wǒ na
IG: you ask me MOD

BT: Are you asking me?
TT1: What's it to you? (mood type: interrogative: wh-)
TT2: Who, me? (mood type: interrogative: wh-)

Example 2.21 (adapted from Lao 1999: 14–15, 2004: 18–19)

ST: 你 要 怎么 着? (interrogative: elemental)
PY: nǐ yào zěn me zhāo
IG: you want how VPART
BT: What do you want to do?
TT1: You want to start something? (declarative)
TT2: What do you think you're doing? (imperative: interrogative: wh-)

Example 2.22 (adapted from Lao 1999: 12–13, 2004: 18–19)

ST: 跟 洋人 干 去, (mood type: imperative: jussive)
PY: gēn yáng rén gàn qù
IG: with foreigners fight CV
BT: Fight with the foreigners.
TT1: why don't you take on the foreigners? (mood type: interrogative: wh-)
TT2: try the foreigners! (mood type: imperative: jussive)

One mood shift is found in the few lines addressed to Master Ma – a villain relying on foreigners' patronage (see Example 2.23). Being totally unaware of who Master Ma is, Master Chang uses an imperative in the ST to implore Master Ma to make some judgments for what Erdez has done. In TT1, instead of translating the imperative equivalently, the translator has rendered it as an interrogative: wh- to convert the speech function of "command" into "question." The translator of TT2, however, maintains the equivalence both in mood and speech function, except for adding a bound clause.

Example 2.23 (adapted from Lao 1999: 16–17, 2004: 20–21)

ST: 您 给 评评理! (mood type: imperative: jussive)
PY: nín gěi píng píng lǐ
IG: you (HON) CV judge
BT: Please judge this!
TT1: Who do you think's in the right? (mood type: interrogative: wh-)
TT2: Please tell us (mood type: imperative: jussive)
who you think was right. (mood type: bound)

2.2.5   *Mood analysis of Qin Zhongyi's lines*

As an enterprising entrepreneur in the late Qing Dynasty in China, Qin Zhongyi is a rich man who owns various real estates, including the house that is used as Wang Lifa's teahouse. He is ambitious and tries to save the empire by developing industry. Therefore, one of his plans is to take back the teahouse, sell off his farmland, and build a factory. In addition, he is tactful in socializing with Eunuch Pang, whom he dislikes and is in conflict with. This contradiction, however, is not only due to their personalities but is also a result of the clashes between the different classes they each belong to (Lan 2007; Yang 2007).

Throughout Act One of the ST, Qin Zhongyi mostly interacts with two characters, i.e. Wang Lifa and Eunuch Pang. Many declaratives are addressed to Wang Lifa in order to inquire about the house, to express his desire to increase the house rent, to state his intention to take back the teahouse, and to explain his plans to build a factory. While addressing Eunuch Pang, declaratives are only used for greeting purposes by Qin Zhongyi. Despite the fact that he and Eunuch Pang are totally at odds with each other, he still shows him respect and flatters him.

Imperatives in the ST, on the other hand, are addressed to Wang Lifa to decline his flattering and to warn him not to refuse to pay the increased rent. However, in addressing Tang the Oracle, imperatives are used to turn him out of the teahouse. As for the only imperative addressed to Eunuch Pang, it is used to depreciate Master Qin himself and to praise Eunuch Pang. In the two TTs, most mood shifts are found in the clauses addressed to Wang Lifa, while those addressed to other characters are translated equivalently in terms of mood type. However, with a small number of such shifts found in the data, no certain tendency of such shifts is found. According to Example 2.24, an imperative in the ST is translated as a declarative in TT1, informing Wang Lifa the futility in flattering Qin Zhongyi. In Example 2.25, both translators have rendered an imperative as a declarative. In this way, the threat of taking back the teahouse in the ST is stated in different ways. In Example 2.26, a minor clause is translated as an imperative: jussive in TT1, revealing that Qin is trying to stop the conversation.

Example 2.24 (adapted from Lao 1999: 30–31, 2004: 32–33)

ST: 可是，用 不 着 奉承 我！(mood type: imperative: jussive)
PY: kě shì, yòng bù zháo fèng chéng wǒ
IG: but need NEG VPART flatter me
BT: But you do not need to flatter me!
TT1: But you'll get nothing by playing up to me. (mood type: declarative)
TT2: But don't make such a fuss. (mood type: imperative: jussive)

Example 2.25 (adapted from Lao 1999: 32–33, 2004: 32–33)

ST: 哼，等 着 吧，(mood type: imperative: jussive)
PY: hèng, děng zhe ba
IG: hum wait VPART MOD
BT: Hum, just wait.
TT1: You'll see. (mood type: declarative)
TT2: You just wait, (mood type: declarative)

Example 2.26 (adapted from Lao 1999: 38–39, 2004: 36–37)

ST: 好 啦, (mood type: minor)
PY: hǎo la
IG: OK MOD
BT: OK,
TT1: Oh, forget it. (mood type: imperative: jussive)
TT2: All right, (mood type: minor)

2.2.6 Mood analysis of Kang Liu's lines

Kang Liu is a poor peasant from the outskirts of Beijing who has to sell his daughter to a monster like Eunuch Pang to be able to feed himself and pay his rent. He is a tragic character who helps depict the tragic atmosphere of the era and create a sense of desolation in the play (Huo 1983).

In terms of the mood distribution in the ST, Kang Liu addresses all his declaratives to Pock-Mark Liu and his daughter Kang Shunz. When the declaratives are addressed to Pock-Mark Liu, they are used to negotiate the issue concerning the sale of his daughter and, later, to explain why Shunz fainted on seeing the monstrous face of Eunuch Pang. For the declaratives addressed to Kang Shunz, they are either used to apologize for selling her or to explain the reason for sending her away. Moreover, the interrogatives in the ST are all addressed to Pock-Mark Liu to negotiate the price of the girl and to inquire about the person whom the girl is being sold to.

In the ST, Kang Liu contributes a very small amount of imperatives (see Table 2.5). Only two imperatives are found (see Example 2.27), which are addressed to Kang Shunz, asking her to accept her miserable fate. In TT1, the first imperative is translated as a declarative in which the speech function of "command" in the ST has been changed to "statement." Thus, the command to let Shunz accept her fate has become a statement used to assert Kang Liu's predicament. For the second imperative in the ST, though the mood type remains unchanged in TT1, the experiential meaning of the lexis "积 德" (PY: jī dé; IG: accumulate fate) has become different – this can be regarded as an error in translation.[2]

Example 2.27 (adapted from Lao 1999: 52–53, 2004: 48–49)

ST: 你 呀, 顺子，认 命 吧, (mood type: imperative: jussive)
PY: nǐ ya, shùn zi, rèn mìng ba
IG: you MOD Shunz accept fate MOD
BT: You, Shunz, accept your fate,
积 德 吧！(mood type: imperative: jussive)
PY: jī dé ba
IG: accumulate virtue MOD
BT: accumulate your virtue!
TT1: There's no other way. (mood type: declarative)

Please don't make things difficult. (mood type: imperative: jussive)
TT2: Shunz, accept your fate (mood type: imperative: jussive)
and have pity on us! (mood type: imperative: jussive)

Besides, we note that Kang Liu has contributed the largest number of minor clauses in the data (nine minor clauses in total, which constitutes 25% of Kang Liu's contribution, see Table 2.5). These minor clauses are mostly Vocatives used to draw the attention of the addressees, such as "顺子" (PY: shùn zi; IG: Shunz), "姑娘" (PY: gū niang; IG: daughter), and "刘爷" (PY: liú ye; IG: Master Liu), or interjections that express his vexation, such as "唉！" (PY: ai; IG: alas).

In the TTs, especially in TT1, we find several examples of interrogatives and imperatives translated as declaratives (see Examples 2.28 and 2.29). As seen in Example 2.28, the biassed type of polar interrogative is a rhetorical question, whereas both translators have chosen to translate it as declaratives, thus stating Kang Liu's difficult situation in a more direct way.

Example 2.28 (adapted from Lao 1999: 18–19, 2004: 22–23)

ST: 那 不 是 因为 乡下 种地的 都 没 法子 混 了 吗？(mood type: interrogative: polar: biassed)
PY: nà bú shì yīn wéi xiāng xià zhòng dì de dōu méi fǎ zi hùn le ma
IG: that NEG be because countryside peasant all have (NEG) way get by ASP MOD
BT: Isn't that because peasants in the countryside all have no way to get by?
TT1: It's because it's impossible for us peasants (mood type: declarative) to get by these days. (mood type: bound)
TT2: We peasants can't live any more. (mood type: declarative)

Moreover, in the TTs, especially TT1, various declaratives and wh- interrogatives tend to be translated as yes/no interrogatives. As shown in Example 2.29, the translator changes a declarative to a yes/no interrogative but retains Kang Liu's accusation and condemnation. In Example 2.30, the mood type is changed from interrogative: wh- to interrogative: yes/no in TT1, as the incomplete clause in the ST is interpreted differently by the two translators. However, the speech function remains equivalent in the TTs. In other words, the three clauses in the ST and both TTs are all questions that express Kang Liu's surprise and sadness on hearing that his daughter is going to marry a eunuch.

Example 2.29 (adapted from Lao 1999: 20–21, 2004: 22–23)

ST: 我 就 不 是 人！(mood type: declarative)
PY: wǒ jiù bú shì rén
IG: I VADV NEG be man
BT: I am then not a man!
TT1: then, could I call myself a man? (mood type: interrogative: yes/no)
TT2: then I'd be a beast! (mood type: declarative)

Example 2.30 (adapted from Lao 1999: 22–23, 2004: 24–25)

ST: 自 古 以来, 哪 有 . . . (mood type: interrogative: elemental)
PY: zì gǔ yǐ lái, nǎ yǒu
IG: since ancient since, where have
BT: Since ancient times, where could . . .
TT1: Has there ever been, from earliest times? (mood type: interrogative: yes/no)
TT2: But who's ever heard of such a thing . . . ? (mood type: interrogative: wh-)

2.2.7 Mood analysis of Master Song's lines

According to the dramatis personae provided by Lao She, Master Song is a "timid and talkative" man (Lao 1999: 13). He is a Manchurian who lives on the subsidy provided by the empire and never does any labor to earn a living. As a regular customer of Wang Lifa's teahouse, he hangs around with his birdcage and chats with other customers. He is timid in that he dares not to speak to Erdez during the fight. However, he is also generous in that he volunteers to pay for the teacup that got broken during the fight between Master Chang and Erdez.

In the ST, most of his imperatives are addressed to Tubby Huang, an underworld boss, to invite him to say a few kind words to the two secret agents in order to save him from getting in trouble. There is another imperative that is addressed to Wang Lifa to ask him to look after his bird while he is away. In addition, Master Song's interrogatives reflect his talkative personality. In this way, he inquires about the turbulence in the backyard, the job of Erdez, Pock-Mark Liu's income for selling a girl, as well as the reason for the fight in the inner courtyard (Feng 2007; Huang 2007).

In TT1, the polar interrogatives in the ST tend to be translated as declaratives (see Examples 2.31, 2.32, and 2.33). These interrogatives are all found in casual conversations rather than being used to challenge the addressees. However, in TT2, this mood type is often translated equivalently, as shown in Examples 2.31 and 2.32. There are also exceptions (see Example 2.33), according to which the polar interrogative is translated as a minor clause and a tagged declarative in TT2. We find moodtags or interjections like "eh" that function similar to a moodtag added in the TTs (see Example 2.33). The use of "eh" in TT1 is a preferred choice of the translator, who adds seven interjections in TT1 to translate the polar interrogatives in the ST.

Example 2.31 (adapted from Lao 1999: 12–13, 2004: 16–17)

ST: 好象 又 有 事儿 ? (mood type: interrogative: polar: biassed)
PY: hǎo xiàng yòu yǒu shì er
IG: seem again have matter
BT: Is there trouble again?
TT1: [ø: It] Looks like trouble again. (mood type: declarative)
TT2: [ø: Is there] Trouble again? (mood type: interrogative: yes/no)

Example 2.32 (adapted from Lao 1999: 22–23, 2004: 26–27)

ST: 这 号 生意 又 不 小 吧? (mood type: interrogative: polar: biassed)
PY: zhèi hào shēng yì yòu bù xiǎo ba
IG: this kind business again NEG small MOD
BT: Is this business not small?
TT1: I expect (mood type: declarative)
you're making a bit on this deal? (mood type: bound)
TT2: [ø: Is it] Another big deal? (mood type: interrogative: yes/no)

Example 2.33 (adapted from Lao 1999: 12–13, 2004: 16–17)

ST: 我 说 这 位 爷，您 是 营 里 当差的 吧? (mood type: interrogative:
polar: biassed)
PY: wǒ shuō zhèi wèi yé, nín shì yíng lǐ dāng chāi de ba
IG: I say this MEAS sir, you (HON) be camp in officer MOD
BT: Sir, are you an official from the camp?
TT1: Well, sir, I'd guess (mood type: declarative)
that you're from the Wrestling Academy, eh? (mood type: bound)
TT2: Excuse me, sir, (mood type: minor)
you serve in the Imperial Wrestlers, don't you? (mood type: declarative:
tagged: reversed polarity)

2.2.8 *Mood analysis of Eunuch Pang's lines*

In the play, Eunuch Pang comes onto the stage only toward the end of Act One. In addition, among all the characters, he has the highest social status, which only Qin Zhongyi can be compared with, as Pang and Qin represent the traditional ideas and the reforming ideas respectively. That is also the reason that leads to their conflict (Tong 2007). During the play, Eunuch Pang comes to the teahouse to buy a wife and to meet the girl to be sold (Kang Shunz) despite the fact that a eunuch never needs to get married. It is in this way that the tragic story of the Kang family is presented.

In the analysis of the ST, it is found that Eunuch Pang uses declaratives to comment on state affairs as well as Qin's business. He uses interrogatives to enquire where Pock-Mark Liu is and to negotiate the price of Kang Shunz. Besides this, three rhetorical questions are found, all of which are polar interrogatives of the biassed type that realize the speech function of "statement," such as "[ø: 您 太 客 气 了 吧？" (PY: nín tài kè qi le ba; IG: you [HON] too modest ASP MOD). Despite his high social status, only three imperatives are found in his lines in the ST. Two are of the jussive type and are used to assure Tang the Oracle and invite Tubby Huang to the wedding respectively; one is of the suggestive type and is addressed to Qin Zhongyi in order to openly argue with him.

In the TTs, though different kinds of mood shift are found, there is a tendency that both translators prefer to render imperatives and polar interrogatives as declaratives (see Examples 2.34, 2.35, and 2.36). Example 2.34 is Eunuch Pang's suggestion to Qin Zhongyi, which is realized as an imperative: suggestive. Example 2.35 is a polar interrogative, which serves as Eunuch Pang's reassurance to Tang the Oracle. Example 2.36 is an imperative: jussive, which functions as an invitation to Tubby Huang. Such clauses have the potential to be translated as declaratives, especially in TT1. By doing so, the translators face another choice, i.e. whether to add a moodtag or not. In Examples 2.35 and 2.36, we find that moodtags are added by reversing the order of Subject and Finite as well as reversing the polarity. In this way, the speaker, Eunuch Pang, invites the addressees to give their responses.

Example 2.34 (adapted from Lao 1999: 40–41, 2004: 40–41)

ST: 咱们 就 八 仙 过 海, (mood type: imperative: suggestive)
PY: zán men jiù bā xiān guò hǎi
IG: we VADV eight deity cross sea
BT: Let's then be like eight deities that cross the sea,
TT1: [ø: It is] Like the Eight Immortals crossing the sea, (mood type: declarative)
TT2: Let's both try our best, (mood type: imperative: suggestive)

Example 2.35 (adapted from Lao 1999: 44–45, 2004: 42–43)

ST: 还 能 不 搜查搜查 谭嗣同 的 余党 吗？(mood type: interrogative: polar: biassed)
PY: hái néng bù sōu chá sōu chá tán sì tóng de yú dǎng ma
IG: yet can NEG look for Tan Sitong SUB remnant follower MOD
BT: Can't they search for Tan Sitong's remnant followers?
TT1: They're doubtless looking for Tan Sitong's remnant followers, aren't they? (mood type: declarative: tagged: reversed polarity)
TT2: They have to nose out Tan Sitong's supporters, don't they? (mood type: declarative: tagged: reversed polarity)

Example 2.36 (adapted from Lao 1999: 50–51, 2004: 48–49)

ST: 等 吃 喜酒 吧！(mood type: imperative: jussive)
PY: děng chī xǐ jiǔ ba
IG: wait for eat wedding wine MOD
BT: Wait for the wine at the wedding party!
TT1: You'll come to the banquet, won't you? (mood type: declarative: tagged: reversed polarity)
TT2: You'll be invited to the banquet! (mood type: declarative)

2.2.9 Mood analysis of Tang the Oracle's lines

Tang the Oracle is a professional fortuneteller who looks for customers in the teahouse. Because Tang never pays for the tea and is a drug addict, Wang Lifa is always trying to drive him out of the teahouse. In terms of Tang's free clauses in the ST, only declaratives and imperatives are found, which means that no inter-rogative clause is used. His declaratives are addressed to Wang Lifa, Qin Zhongyi, and Eunuch Pang, either to ask for a cup of tea, to try to find a customer for himself, or to give an excuse for staying in the teahouse. His imperatives are all addressed to Wang Lifa to ask the manager of the teahouse to give him some tea for free.

Despite the fact that few imperatives are used by Tang the Oracle in the ST, in the TTs, an even smaller number of this mood type is found. In Example 2.37, both translators have translated the imperative of the oblative type as declaratives, but the speech function of the two clauses is still "offer," which remains unchanged.

Example 2.37 (adapted from Lao 1999: 8–9, 2004: 14–15)

ST: 我 就 先 给 您 相相面 吧！(mood type: imperative: oblative)
PY: wǒ jiù xiān gěi nín xiàng xiàng miàn ba
IG: I VADV first CV you (HON) tell fortune MOD
BT: Let me first tell you your fortune.
TT1: and I'll tell you your fortune. (mood type: declarative)
TT2: and I'll tell your fortune for you. (mood type: declarative)

While translating the two declaratives in Example 2.38, the translator of TT1 has added two imperatives (one jussive and one oblative). Also, by adding "let me see your palm," an additional offer of providing services to Wang Lifa is indicated. However, different from TT1's translator, the translator of TT2 has translated the mood type in this example equivalently and has combined the two declarative clauses into one clause.

Example 2.38 (adapted from 1999: 8–9, 2004: 14–15)

ST: 手相 奉送，(mood type: declarative)
PY: shǒu xiàng fèng sòng
IG: palm-reading for free
BT: Palm-reading is for free
不 取 分文！(mood type: declarative)
PY: bù qǔ fēn wén
IG: NEG charge any money
BT: I won't charge any money!
TT1: Come on, (mood type: imperative: jussive)
let me see your palm – (mood type: imperative: oblative)
[ø: It] won't cost you a cent. (mood type: declarative)
TT2: With palm-reading thrown in, it won't cost you a copper! (mood type: declarative)

Though no interrogative is found in the ST, one occurrence of wh- interrogative is added in TT2, which is translated from a bound clause (see Example 2.39). In addition, the declarative clause in the ST is omitted. In this case, Tang the Oracle addresses the question directly to Wang Lifa to enquire about the turbulence in the street.

Example 2.39 (adapted from Lao 1999: 44–45, 2004: 42–43)

ST: [ø: 我] 不 知道 (mood type: declarative)
PY: wǒ bù zhī dào
IG: I NEG know
BT: I don't know
[ø: 街 上] 是 怎么 回 事! (mood type: bound)
PY: jiē shàng shì zěn me huí shì
IG: street in be how MEAS going-on
BT: what is going on in the street?
TT1: I don't know (mood type: declarative)
what's going on. (mood type: bound)
TT2: What's happening? (mood type: interrogative: wh-)

2.2.10   Mood analysis of Erdez's lines

Erdez is an imperial wrestler whose responsibility is to safeguard Beijing. He comes to the teahouse to settle a dispute, and he regards himself as a powerful and prestigious person. Therefore, Master Chang's comment on the dispute, i.e. "they won't come into blows," irritates him and nearly results in a fight between him and Master Chang. However, on hearing Master Ma's shout to him,[3] he calms down immediately and pretends to be friendly, as Master Ma has a higher social status than him (Li 2007).

In the ST, Erdez is depicted as a thug or a hatchet man. On the one hand, he challenges and threatens Master Chang by using a large number of interrogatives. On the other hand, he tries his best to be humble by using several declaratives and one interrogative to greet Master Ma. He even promises to pay for Master Ma's tea. Some mood shifts are found in the TTs. As shown in Example 2.40, the imperative and the bound clause in the ST are translated as a minor clause in TT1, with an extra meaning of cursing or condemning the foreigners added in TT1 to depict the brutality of Erdez. However, in TT2, the translator has chosen to retain the imperative mood equivalently.

Example 2.40 (adapted from Lao 1999: 14–15, 2004: 18–19)

ST: 甭 说 (mood type: imperative: jussive)
PY: béng shuō
IG: NEG say
BT: Don't say
[ø: 我] 打 洋人 不 打, (mood type: bound)
PY: wǒ dǎ yáng rén bù dǎ
IG: I beat foreigner NEG beat
BT: I beat the foreigners or not
TT1: To hell with the foreigners, (mood type: minor)
TT2: Leave the foreigners out of this! (mood type: imperative: jussive)

In Example 2.41, the elemental interrogative used by Erdez to threaten Master Chang is translated as a declarative, which serves as a response to Master Chang's question – "You want to start something?" In TT2, however, the translator has left this clause untranslated, thus leaving Master Chang's question, i.e. "What do you think you're doing?" unanswered. As a matter of fact, before they start a fight, the question does not need an answer.

Example 2.41 (adapted from Lao 1999: 14–15, 2004: 18–19)

ST: [ø: 我 想] 怎么 着？(mood type: interrogative: elemental)
PY: wǒ xiǎng zěn me zhāo
IG: I want to how VPART
BT: What do I want?
TT1: [ø: I want to] start something? (mood type: declarative)
TT2: (omitted)

In addition, polar interrogatives by Erdez tend to be translated as declaratives (see Examples 2.42 and 2.43). In Example 2.42, the two declaratives in both TTs clearly state Erdez's reason for starting a fight. The translator of TT1 has chosen to use an interjection "eh?" to raise a question. In Example 2.43, the question addressed to Master Ma is changed to declaratives in both TTs to help Erdez speak in an indirect way, while the Subject of the two indicative clauses has also been changed from "您" (PY: nín; IG: you [HON]) in the ST to "I" in the TTs, which is a shift made in the system of SUBJECT PERSON.

Example 2.42 (adapted from Lao 1999: 14–15, 2004: 18–19)

ST: 我 碰 不 了 洋人，(mood type: declarative)
PY: wǒ pèng bù liǎo yáng rén
IG: I touch NEG ASP foreigner
BT: I don't touch the foreigners
[ø: 我] 还 碰 不 了 你 吗？(mood type: interrogative: polar: biassed)
PY: wǒ hái pèng bù liǎo nǐ ma
IG: I then touch NEG ASP you MOD
BT: Don't I touch you?
TT1: So, I can't handle the foreigners, eh? (mood type: declarative)
Well, I can surely handle you. (mood type: declarative)
TT2: Perhaps I don't touch the foreigners, (mood type: declarative)
but I'll give you one of me touches. (mood type: declarative)
I will! (mood type: declarative)

Example 2.43 (adapted from Lao 1999: 14–15, 2004: 18–19)

ST: 喝， 马五爷，您 在 这儿 哪？(mood type: interrogative: polar: biassed)
PY: he, mǎ wǔ ye, nín zài zhè er na
IG: oh Master Ma you (HON) CV here MOD

BT: Oh, Master Ma, are you here?
TT1: Fifth Elder Ma, I didn't know (mood type: declarative)
you were here. (mood type: bound)
TT2: sir, I never see (mood type: declarative)
you sitting there. (mood type: bound)

2.2.11   *Mood analysis of Song Enz and Wu Xiangz's lines*

Song Enz and Wu Xiangz are two of the old-fashioned secret agents commonly referred to as "the two grey gowns" because of the clothes they wear (Ren 2007). They hide themselves in a corner of the teahouse and are ready to arrest those who dare to openly discuss state affairs. In the playscript, they only interact with Master Chang and Master Song at the end of Act One while trying to arrest these two regular customers.[4]

In the ST, we find that the amount of interrogatives and imperatives contributed by the two characters is large (see Table 2.5). These clauses congruently realize the speech functions of "question" and "command," which help Lao She to create a terrifying atmosphere in the teahouse as well as in the era where the events take place. In the TTs, similar to the lines of the other characters, there is also a tendency of translating the polar interrogatives as declaratives and to occasionally add moodtags. The motivation for these shifts is not to speak indirectly to the addressee, but the opposite, i.e. to be direct, forceful, active, and aggressive (cf. Figure 2.3). In Example 2.44, a polar interrogative is translated as a declarative in the TTs, with no moodtag added, whereas in Example 2.45, the translator of TT1 has added a moodtag to give a further warning to Master Chang, even though there is no Chinese equivalent like "是 吧" (PY: shì ba; IG: be MOD) or "是 吗" (PY: shì ma; IG: be MOD) in the ST.

Example 2.44 (adapted from Lao 1999: 48–49, 2004: 44–45)

ST: 你 还 想 拒 捕 吗？(mood type: interrogative: polar: biassed)
PY: nǐ hái xiǎng jù bǔ ma
IG: you even want to resist arrest MOD
BT: Do you even want to resist arrest?
TT1: So you're going to resist arrest as well? (mood type: declarative)
TT2: So you're resisting arrest? (mood type: declarative)

Example 2.45 (adapted from Lao 1999: 46–47, 2004: 44–45)

ST: 你 听见 了？(mood type: interrogative: polar: biassed)
PY: nǐ tīng jiàn le
IG: you hear ASP
BT: Did you hear him?
TT1: You heard him, didn't you? (mood type: declarative: tagged: reversed
   polarity)
TT2: You heard him? (mood type: declarative)

2.2.12 Mood analysis of Li San's lines

Li San is an experienced waiter at Yutai Teahouse. He is hard-working, kind-hearted, and is very helpful to Wang Lifa, who works as the manager at a young age. Because of his job in the teahouse, he has to talk less and work more onstage. According to Li Xiang (2007), the actor who plays Li San in the performances by Beijing People's Art Theatre, this character is indispensable to the performance. To carry on the performance and to create the environment of a teahouse, he has to provide a lot of services to the customers, such as adding water to tea cups, looking after the customers' birds or crickets, and greeting the customers that just come in. He talks little, not because he has no opinion or attitude but because of his status as a waiter, which makes him unwilling to state his views in public.

In the ST, the only three characters Li San interacts with are the old man selling small wares, Master Song, and the little girl being sold by her mother. His declaratives are mostly used to discuss the fight in the inner courtyard. His imperatives are all used to drive the old man and the little girl outside, to offer noodles to the little girl, and to advise Master Song not to discuss the fight. Only one interrogative clause is found in the data, which is used to inquire about the old man's age.

Similar to Wang Lifa's lines, Li San's imperatives and wh- interrogatives also tend to be translated as declaratives in both TTs. As a result of these shifts in mood type, Li San tends to speak more indirectly and implicitly in the TTs (see Figure 2.3). In Example 2.46, both translators have translated the imperative of the jussive subtype as a declarative. We can note that Li San uses the honorific "您" (PY: nín; IG: you [HON]) rather than "你" (PY: nǐ; IG: you) to address the old man. By the same token, in Examples 2.47 and 2.48, an imperative of the suggestive subtype and a wh- interrogative in the ST are translated as declaratives for the same reason of conveying indirectness and implicitness. In both cases, changes are made in terms of speech function, as a result of which Li San does not directly question or command the addressees in the TTs.

Example 2.46 (adapted from Lao 1999: 28–29, 2004: 30–31)

ST: 老大爷，您外边遛遛吧! (mood type: imperative: jussive)
PY: lǎo dà ye, nín wài biān liù liù ba
IG: old uncle you (HON) outside walk MOD
BT: Old uncle, please take a walk outside!
TT1: Hey, grandpa, you'd better try somewhere else. (mood type: declarative)
TT2: Now, old uncle, [ø: you'd] better try somewhere else. (mood type: declarative)

Example 2.47 (adapted from Lao 1999: 28–29, 2004: 30–31)

ST: 唉，咱们还是少说话好, (mood type: imperative: suggestive)
PY: ai, zán men hái shì shǎo shuō huà hǎo
IG: alas we rather be less talk good
BT: Alas, let's talk less.

TT1: The less we say the better. (mood type: declarative)
TT2: Well, [ø: we'd] better not go into it. (mood type: declarative)

Example 2.48 (adapted from Lao 1999: 28–29, 2004: 30–31)

ST: 老 大爷 您 高寿 啦？(mood type: interrogative: elemental)
PY: lǎo dà ye nín gāo shòu la
IG: old uncle you (HON) what age MOD
BT: Old uncle, what is your age?
TT1: Grandpa, you must be well on in years. (mood type: declarative)
TT2: Old uncle, you must be well on in years. (mood type: declarative)

2.2.13 Analysis of moodtags

According to the mood analysis, no moodtag is found in the ST, while a small number of moodtags are added to the TTs. In terms of the total occurrence, six and nine moodtags are found in both TTs respectively. The number of moodtags is small in TT1, because the translator prefers to use "eh?" at the end of declaratives, which functions similarly as moodtags (see Examples 2.13, 2.33, 2.42). In the TTs, we find that the moodtags are translated from declaratives, yes/no interrogatives, and imperatives in the ST (see Figure 2.4), among which polar interrogatives are the primary source for moodtags in both TTs. Some examples suggest that the translators add moodtags whenever they think it necessary for the speaker to invite a verbal response from the addressee.

In the TTs, most moodtags are added to declaratives, with only one moodtag added to an imperative. According to Example 2.49, the imperative is translated as three clauses (one declarative and two bound clauses) in TT1, while in TT2, the mood type is translated equivalently, and a moodtag is added to request the response of the addresses and also to prevent the customers from discussing state affairs.

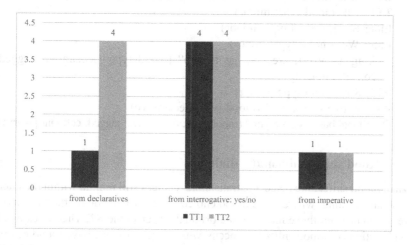

Figure 2.4 Moodtags translated from different mood types in the ST

Example 2.49 (adapted from Lao 1999: 44–45, 2004: 42–43)

ST: 诸位 主顾，咱们 还 是 莫 谈 国 事 吧! (mood type: imperative: suggestive)

PY: zhū wèi zhǔ gù, zán men hái shì mò tán guó shì ba

IG: fellow customers we rather be NEG discuss state affair MOD

BT: Customers, we'd rather not discuss state affairs.

TT1: Gentlemen, I don't think (mood type: declarative)

it's a good idea to (mood type: bound)

discuss state affairs. (mood type: bound)

TT2: Gentlemen, let's leave off discussing affairs of state, shall we? (mood type: imperative: suggestive: tagged: constant polarity)

The tagged clauses can also be further differentiated in terms of polarity, viz. the reversed polarity (the unmarked choice) and the constant polarity (the marked choice). In most cases, both translators choose the reversed polarity for the moodtags. Quantitatively, one choice of constant polarity is found in TT1, and two such choices are found in TT2. As shown in Example 2.50, both translators have chosen to expand the polar interrogative into several clauses, and they have also chosen the tagged declarative and constant polarity. In other words, the moodtag for the declaratives is "are you" instead of "aren't you," as the character – Tubby Huang – only wants to greet the two secret agents, and no answer to the moodtag is required.

Example 2.50 (adapted from Lao 1999: 50–51, 2004: 46–47)

ST: 哟，宋 爷，吴 爷，二 位 办 案 哪？(mood type: interrogative: polar: biassed)

PY: yo, sòng yé, wú yé, èr wèi bàn àn na

IG: yo Song master Wu master two MEAS handle case MOD

BT: Yo, Master Song, Master Wu, are you handling a case?

TT1: Yo! (mood type: minor)

Elder Song. (mood type: minor)

Elder Wu. (mood type: minor)

Making an arrest, are you, gentlemen? (mood type: declarative: tagged: constant polarity)

TT2: So! (mood type: minor)

It's you two gentlemen! (mood type: declarative)

On official business, are you? (mood type: declarative: tagged: constant polarity)

2.3   Mood shift in dramatic dialogue

When mood shifts take place, the translators' choices still remain within the interpersonal meaning, whereas the mood choices in the TTs made by the translators are different from those made by the original writer in the ST. Theoretically, all combinations of mood shifts may occur, while in practice, we have found certain combinations with varied frequencies. Table 2.6 tabulates the types of mood shift

Table 2.6 Different types of mood shift in the analysis of dramatic dialogue

	Types of mood shift		*freq. in TT1*	*freq. in TT2*
change of mood type	constant speech function	declarative → interrogative: elemental	3	1
		declarative → interrogative: polar	2	0
		declarative → bound	6	2
		imperative → declarative	9	13
		imperative → interrogative: elemental	2	2
		imperative → interrogative: polar	0	2
		interrogative: elemental → declarative	4	3
		interrogative: elemental → interrogative: polar	2	1
		interrogative: elemental → bound	1	0
		interrogative: polar → declarative	16	16
		interrogative: polar → interrogative: elemental	4	4
		interrogative: polar → bound	1	0
	converted speech function	declarative → imperative (statement → offer)	1	0
		declarative → imperative (statement → command)	6	7
		declarative → interrogative: elemental (statement → question)	0	2
		declarative → minor	1	1
		imperative → declarative (command → statement)	11	8
		imperative → interrogative: elemental (command → question)	4	1
		imperative → interrogative: polar (command → question)	1	0
		imperative → minor	3	1
		interrogative: polar → declarative (question → statement)	10	7
		interrogative: polar → imperative (question → statement)	1	1
		interrogative: polar → minor	1	2
		interrogative: elemental → declarative (question → statement)	1	0
		interrogative: elemental → declarative (question → command)	0	2
		interrogative: elemental → imperative (question → command)	0	1
		bound → declarative	1	1
		bound → imperative	0	1
		bound → interrogative: elemental	0	1
		minor → imperative	1	2
		minor → declarative	2	5
clause addition			17	21
clause omission			10	11
Total			121	119

found in the data, including the change of mood type, clause addition, and clause omission. Furthermore, the changes of mood type are differentiated according to the speech functions involved, i.e. whether the speech functions in the ST and TTs are constant or converted.

The following examples (Examples 2.51 and 2.52) illustrate mood shifts in relation to the change of speech function. Both examples involve mood shifts from imperative to declarative. On the one hand, in Example 2.51, the speech function remains unchanged, and only change of mood type is found. The clauses in the ST and the TTs all reveal Pock-Mark Liu's insistence to ask Master Song to keep the tiny watch. On the other hand, in Example 2.52, the mood type and the speech function in TT1 are both changed, with the speech function converted from "command" to "statement." However, despite the change of speech function, the declarative in TT1 still serves as Qin Zhongyi's response to Wang Lifa, which is a decline to Wang's compliments.

Example 2.51 (adapted from Lao 1999: 26–27, 2004: 28–29)

ST: 松二爷，留下这个表吧，(mood type: imperative: jussive; speech function: command)

PY: sōng èr yé, liú xià zhèi ge biǎo ba

IG: Master Song keep CV this watch MOD

BT: Master Song, keep this watch!

TT1: Second Elder Song, you'd better hang onto that watch. (mood type: declarative; speech function: command)

TT2: Master Song, you really ought to keep this watch. (mood type: declarative; speech function: command)

Example 2.52 (adapted from Lao 1999: 30–31, 2004: 32–33)

ST: 可是，用不着奉承我! (mood type: imperative: jussive; speech function: command)

PY: kě shì, yòng bù zháo fèng chéng wǒ

IG: but need NEG VPART flatter me

BT: But don't flatter me!

TT1: But you'll get nothing by playing up to me. (mood type: declarative; speech function: statement)

TT2: But don't make such a fuss. (mood type: imperative: jussive; speech function: command)

According to Table 2.6, a similar number of the total mood shifts is found in TT1 and TT2. Three kinds of shift contribute to the largest proportion, i.e. the shift from imperative to declarative, and the shift from interrogative: polar to declarative as well as the increase of clauses (clause addition).

Mood shifts from imperative to declarative are mostly found in the lines of Wang Lifa, Pock-Mark Liu, and Li San. These clauses are addressed to those who are superior, such as Wang Lifa to Qin Zhongyi, Pock-Mark Liu to Master Song and Eunuch Pang, and Li San to Master Song. Whenever these characters are speaking to their customers or potential clients, such mood shifts are likely to be found, which may even lead to the change in speech function (see Example 2.53). In addition, these shifts explain why the frequencies of imperatives in the two TTs are smaller than that of the ST.

Example 2.53 (adapted from Lao 1999: 18–19, 2004: 20–21)

ST: [ø: 咱们] 待会儿 再 算 吧! (mood type: imperative: suggestive; speech function: command)
PY: zán men dāi huì er zài suàn ba
IG: we later then settle MOD
BT: Let's settle this later.
TT1: we'll square up later. (mood type: declarative; speech function: statement)
TT2: We can settle that later. (mood type: declarative; speech function: statement)

By the same token, the mood shifts from interrogative: polar to declarative are often related to certain characters in the play, especially Pock-Mark Liu, Erdez, Eunuch Pang, Song Enz, and Wu Xiangz. Most of these lines are addressed to persons who have little power in terms of tenor relations, including Pock-Mark Liu to Kang Liu, Eunuch Pang to Pock-Mark Liu, and Song Enz and Wu Xiangz to Master Chang and Master Song. In Example 2.54, Pock-Mark Liu's polar interrogative, which is addressed to Kang Liu, is translated as a declarative in TT2 when Pock-Mark Liu threatens Kang Liu to sell Kang Shunz. The increased frequency of mood shifts from interrogative to declarative also explains why there has been an increase in the amount of polar interrogatives in the TTs.

Example 2.54 (adapted from Lao 1999: 20–21, 2004: 24–25)

ST: 这 不 是 造化 吗 ? (mood type: interrogative: polar: biassed; speech function statement)
PY: zhè bú shì zào hua ma
IG: this NEG be good luck MOD
BT: Isn't that good luck?
TT1: Isn't that good fortune? (mood type: interrogative: yes/no; speech function statement)
TT2: I call that a lucky fate! (mood type: declarative; speech function statement)

Another significant mood shift is the addition of clauses in the TTs. We find that most of the additions are minor clauses, which are either realized by interjections or Vocatives. Most interjections are not found in the ST but are added by the two translators for various purposes. For instance, in TT1, "You!", which is addressed by Erdez to Master Chang, is added to draw Master Chang's attention. In TT2, "Bah!", which is used by Eunuch Pang to address several people beside him, is added to reveal Eunuch Pang's anger after talking to Qin Zhongyi. Moreover, we find that interjections that function as textual Themes in the ST are often translated as minor clauses (see Example 2.55). The translator of TT1 renders the interjection "哟" (PY: yo; IG: oh) as one minor clause; while the translator of TT2 chooses to translate the interjection and the Vocative only, thereby omitting the clause in the ST.

Example 2.55 (adapted from Lao 1999: 50–51, 2004: 48–49)

ST: 哟，老爷 在 这儿 哪？(mood type: interrogative: biassed)
PY: yo, lǎo ye zài zhè er na
IG: oh master CV here MOD
BT: Oh, is my master here?
TT1: Yo! (mood type: minor)
You here too, Elder Pang? (mood type: declarative)
TT2: Ah, Your Excellency! (mood type: minor)

2.4　Summary

In this chapter, we conducted an interpersonal analysis of the mood choices in the dramatic dialogue of *Teahouse*. The analysis of mood was further related to the characterization of the leading characters in *Teahouse*, such as Pock-Mark Liu, Wang Lifa, and Master Chang. Some patterns of change in mood type were then found in the TTs. In addition, we quantified and discussed the various subcategories of the mood shift – one kind of metafunctional translation shifts within the interpersonal metafunction (Matthiessen 2014b). The substitutions of mood type were further categorized in accordance with the translation of the speech functions, i.e. whether the speech functions in the ST are maintained or converted in the TTs. The patterns found in the data were identified and the frequently occurred shifts were discussed.

Some typological similarities and differences between English and Chinese were observed based on the lexicogrammatical analysis of mood:

First, for both languages, the basic choices in the system of MOOD are the same (see Figure 2.2). For a major clause, one can choose among the options of declarative, interrogative, and imperative in both languages. As seen in the data, "他们 在 后院 哪！" (PY: tā men zài hòu yuàn na; IG: they CV back courtyard MOD) – a declarative in the ST is translated as "They're in the inner courtyard" in both TTs, and the equivalence of mood type is maintained.

Second, when choosing the option of polar interrogative in Chinese, a further distinction of biassed and unbiassed subtypes can be made, which can be considered as a systemic difference between the two languages. Therefore, when translating biassed and unbiassed polar interrogatives, trade-offs have to be made in the translations. For instance, "十 两 银子 行 不 行？" (PY: shí liǎng yín zi xíng bù xíng; IG: ten tael silver can NEG can), an unbiassed polar interrogative, is translated as "How about ten taels of silver?" and "Will ten taels of silver do?" – a wh- interrogative and a yes/no interrogative – in both TTs respectively. In another example, a interrogative – "您的 事情 都 顺心 吧？" (PY: nín de shì qing dōu shùn xīn ba; IG: your [HON] thing all satisfactory MOD) is rendered as yes/no interrogatives in the two TTs, viz. "Is business going well?" and "[ø: Is your business] Thriving?"

Third, in the Chinese ST, we often find Subjects being omitted in the clauses. In the TTs, the translators often have to add the Subjects back or choose different Subjects. For instance, in "哥儿们，都 是 街面 上 的 朋友，" (PY: gē er men, dōu shì jiē miàn shàng de péng you; IG: brother, all be street on SUB friend), the Subject "我们" (PY: wǒ men; IG: we) or "咱们" (PY: zán men; IG: we) is omitted. In the two TTs, both translators choose to add the Subject "we," as seen in "Now, brothers, we're all neighbors" and "Surely we can settle this as friends."

Fourth, according to the existing systemic functional descriptions of Chinese (e.g. Halliday & McDonald 2004; Li 2007), there is no Finite in the Mood structure, unlike in English. Thus, the mood type of a clause in Chinese is not determined by the syntagmatic order of Subject and Finite. In the TTs, Finites were unconsciously added by the translators during the translation process.

Fifth, we find the abundant use of modal particles in the Chinese ST, including "吗" (PY: ma), "啦" (PY: la), "吧" (PY: ba), "呢" (PY: ne), "啊" (PY: a), "哪" (PY: na), "呀" (PY: ya), and "嘛" (PY: ma). Some of them signal certain mood types, such as "吗" (PY: ma) in "他 是 这么 说 的 吗？" (PY: tā shì zhè me shuō de ma; IG: he EMPH this say VPART MOD), which marks a polar interrogative in Chinese. Some of them indicate emphasis, such as "啊" (PY: a; IG: MOD) in "二德子，你 威风 啊！" (PY: èr dé zi, nǐ wēi feng a; IG: Erdez you powerful MOD). Some of them help soften the tone, such as "吧" (PY: ba; IG: MOD) in "待会儿 再 算 吧！" (PY: dài huì er zài suàn ba; IG: later then settle MOD). These clause-final particles function in the system of MODAL ASSESSMENT and are found in various languages around the world, such as Japanese in Asia (e.g. Teruya 2004, 2007) and Dagaare in Africa (e.g. Mwinlaaru 2018).

While recreating the interpersonal meaning in translation, translators first choose to interpret the propositions, proposals, and assessments in the source text, then they reenact such interpersonal meanings by using the resources in the target language (Matthiessen 2014b). Based on the lexicogrammatical analysis of mood in this chapter, we can summarize some trade-offs that the translators of the TTs have to face. First, it is not compulsory for translators to achieve the equivalence of mood. They may choose a different mood type to maintain the equivalence semantically, to maintain other modes of meaning, or to depict the characters in a certain way. An awareness of the choices in the system of MOOD will help translators make their choices during the translation process. Second, options in the systems of MODALITY and MOOD TAG will help translators in the reenactment of interpersonal meaning. Third, when adopting a "free" translation strategy, translation shifts may be found in both the lexicogrammatical system of MOOD and the semantic system of SPEECH FUNCTION. The translator will then be operating in a larger environment in terms of stratification, i.e. context (Matthiessen 2001).

Notes

1 Parts of Sections 2.2.1, 2.2.2, and 2.2.3 are published in Wang and Ma (2019). Some revisions have been made in this book.
2 In his study on translation, Halliday (2010) relates linguistic analysis to error analysis, which used to be a popular method in the 1970s (cf. Corder 1967). He holds that error analysis, despite its current unpopularity, is helpful for students of linguistics, as it helps them become conscious of the different dimensions of language.
3 According to Li Yuan (2007), the actor of Erdez Senior and Erdez Junior, Master Ma's shouting of Erdez's name is different in that he calls Erdez directly, while other people will honor him as "Master Erdez."
4 In the performances by Beijing People's Art Theatre, some changes were made in this part. When acting onstage, before Song Enz and Wu Xiangz arrest Master Chang and Master Song, they also interact with Eunuch Pang to greet him and to secretly inform him about the arrest. This plot is added by the director and is not found in the published playscript.

3 Re-presenting textual meaning in dramatic monologue[1]

This chapter reports on findings from the thematic analysis of dramatic monologue. As stated in Section 1.2, all dramatic monologues in *Teahouse* are addressed to the audience by one character named Silly Young, who is a beggar that earns a living by chanting rhythmic storytelling. In Section 3.1, we introduce the concept of theme in SFL. In Section 3.2, we analyze the choices of Theme in the complete dramatic monologue, providing a quantitative profile of the analysis. Section 3.3 then elaborates the Theme shifts found in the analysis and their delicate categories.

3.1 A description of theme in systemic functional terms

Vilém Mathesius (e.g. 1928, 1975) first introduced the concept of theme, which originated from the works on functional sentence perspective (FSP) written by various Prague school scholars (cf. Daneš 1974; Firbas 1964, 1992). Most Prague school scholars have accepted Mathesius' (e.g. 1928, 1975) view, according to which theme is interpreted as "that which is known or at least obvious in the given situation and from which the speaker proceeds" (Firbas 1964: 286). According to this definition, thematic information can be understood from the following two perspectives: "(i) information which is known or obvious in the situation, (ii) information from which the speaker proceeds" (Fries 1995: 1; cf. Fries 1981).

In SFL, Halliday (1967a, 1967b, 1985a) distinguishes between the two notions of theme mentioned earlier by using Given to refer to the already known information (i.e. the first perspective) and by recognizing Theme as "the point of departure of the message" (i.e. the second perspective). Fries (1995) has differentiated these two approaches as "the combining approach" and "the splitting approach." In this way, theme and information have been separated, so that Given and New as well as Theme and Rheme constitute different layers of analysis in SFL. The elements of Given and New consist of the information structures, while Theme and Rheme partly comprise the thematic structure of the clause.

The following definitions of Theme are found in Halliday's works throughout the decades:

1   The Theme is what is being talked about, the point of departure for the clause as message.

(Halliday 1967b: 212)

2   The English clause consists of a "Theme" and a "Rheme." . . . [The Theme] is as it were the peg on which the message is hung. . . . The Theme of the clause is the element which, in English, is put in first position.

(Halliday 1970: 161)

3   The Theme is the element which serves as the point of departure of the message; it is that with which the clause is concerned.

(Halliday 1985a: 38)

4   As a general guide, the Theme can be identified as that element which comes in first position in the clause. . . . The Theme is one element in a particular structural configuration which, taken as a whole, organizes the clause as a message. . . . A message consists of a Theme combined with a Rheme. Within that configuration, the Theme is the starting-point for the message; it is what the clause is going to be about.

(Halliday 1985a: 39)

5   The Theme is the element which serves as the point of departure of the message; it is that which locates and orients the clause within its context.

(Halliday & Matthiessen 2014: 89)

From these definitions, we note that Theme is regarded as a functional unit. It is thus described as "point of departure for the clause as message" (Halliday 1967b: 212) or "peg on which the message is hung" (Halliday 1970: 161). Furthermore, the initial position of Theme is first described in the grammar of English; whereas for other languages, Theme can be realized by other resources, for example, the use of certain particles in Japanese (Teruya 2004, 2007) or affixes in Tagalog (Martin 2004).

Some other distinctions of Theme are made. A Theme can be distinguished as marked or unmarked. In a declarative clause, a topical Theme will be marked if it is anything besides the Subject. If a Theme is the Subject, then it is unmarked. Besides, in one Theme, the first referential element which can either be a participant, circumstance, or process is termed topical Theme. Topical Theme can be preceded by certain optional elements, i.e. textual Themes and interpersonal Themes, whose functions are either textual or interpersonal. In Example 3.1 (see Table 3.1), "But" is the textual Theme, which is realized by a conjunction; "Your Majesty" – a Vocative functions as the interpersonal Theme; "an emperor," realized by a participant, is the topical Theme and is the unmarked type, as it is the

Table 3.1 Example 3.1

But,	Your Majesty,	an emperor	should have seventy-two concubines apart from his official wives.
textual Theme	interpersonal Theme	unmarked topical Theme	Rheme
Given ←			New

Source: Adapted from Lao (1999: 175)

Subject in the declarative clause. In addition, the information structure of the clause is Given ^ New, which means that the Theme falls within the Given, and the New falls within the Rheme.

Descriptions of THEME in Mandarin Chinese have revealed the choices in the system and the different types of Theme (e.g. Halliday & McDonald 2004; Li 2007). According to the existing descriptions, textual Theme, interpersonal Theme, and topical Theme are all found in Chinese. In Section 3.4, we will discuss some similarities and differences in the realizations of the Theme choices.

Thematic analysis has been applied to the analysis of texts of various registers, such as scientific discourse (Halliday 1990), literary discourse (Goatly 1995; Martin 1995), academic discourse (Whittaker 1995), and sports commentary (Ghadessy 1995). Linguists have benefited a great deal from thematic analyses. As Ventola (1995: 85) suggests, "in literary analysis, they [thematic analyses] give insight to the author's style; in language teaching, they provide text-structuring help to novice writers." By adopting different methodologies (be it quantitative, qualitative, or both), these studies have revealed various findings and have several implications. Moreover, instead of being viewed "from below" or "roundabout," it is suggested that the system of THEME has to be viewed "from above" (Halliday 1996), i.e. to be viewed from the perspective of semantics (see Martin 1983; Matthiessen 1995b) in order to interpret motivations for the choices of Theme. In terms of the application of thematic analysis to translation, Baker (1992) highlights the importance of Theme in her classic textbook on translation. Kim and Matthiessen (2015) and Wang (2014) conduct comprehensive reviews from two perspectives: (i) the recreation of textual choices, to what extent are the choices in the target text similar or different to those in the ST; and (ii) the appliability of SFL to translation studies.

3.2 Analysis of Theme in dramatic monologue

Based on previous descriptions of Chinese and English, we know that three types of Theme can be identified in both languages: textual Theme, interpersonal Theme, and topical Theme (see Matthiessen 1995a; Halliday & Matthiessen 2014 for descriptions of English grammar and Halliday & McDonald 2004; Li 2007 for

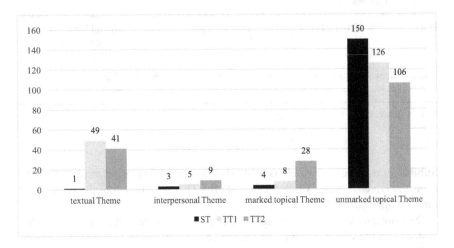

Figure 3.1 Frequency of different types of Theme in the analysis of dramatic monologue

descriptions of Chinese grammar). Figure 3.1 presents the frequency of different types of Theme based on the analysis of dramatic monologue.

3.2.1   Analysis of textual Theme in dramatic monologue

In terms of textual Theme, one is found in the ST (49 in TT1 and 41 in TT2). These textual Themes are all realized by either conjunction, continuative, or conjunctive Adjunct. According to Table 3.2, most textual Themes in the TTs are conjunctions, such as "and," "but," "if," and "when," which are added by the two translators, although there is only one conjunction in the ST, namely "自从" (PY: zì cóng; IG: since). The additions of conjunctions in the TTs reveal the typological differences between Chinese and English, as it is a general feature for Chinese to have fewer conjunctions (Li & Thompson 1981).

Example 3.2 shows how conjunctions, namely "But if" in TT1 and "But" in TT2, are added by the translators. The additions give rise to translation shifts from textual to logical metafunction, which make the implicit textual transitions in the ST explicit. In the Chinese ST, all textual transitions are implicit; hence, readers or the audience would have to make their own inference. However, in both TTs, the translators have added various cohesive conjunctions to make such transitions explicit. The reason behind this is that the Chinese monologue is written in the form of doggerel that seldom contains connectors. According to the couplet style of the storytelling, the numbers of the Chinese characters in two adjacent lines are normally the same. Conjunctions in Chinese, such as "然后" (PY: rán hòu; IG: and), "可是" (PY: kě shì; IG: but), and "因为" (PY: yīn wéi; IG: because) will not only be regarded as redundant but will also destroy the rhythmic pattern in Chinese

Table 3.2 Frequency of textual Theme in the analysis of dramatic monologue

	ST	*TT1*	*TT2*
conjunction	1	48	37
continuative	0	1	3
conjunctive Adjunct	0	0	1
Total	1	49	41

(see Section 5.3.3 for the analysis of mode). Also in Example 3.2, apart from the conjunctions, there is the use of a continuative – "Well" that functions as a textual Theme in TT1.

Example 3.2 (adapted from Lao 1999: 230–231, 2004: 188–189)[2]

ST: 没 有 钱 的 只好 白 瞧 着。
PY: méi yǒu qián de zhǐ hǎo bái qiáo zhe
IG: NEG have money SUB have to NEG look VPART
BT: People without money have to look.
TT1: **But if** you're broke. . . .
Well, watching's free.
TT2: **But** not a crumb for those who cannot pay.

Continuatives and conjunctive Adjuncts that function as textual Themes are not found in the ST, and their frequencies in the TTs are quite small. They are added to the TTs as a result of the translators' preferences. In Example 3.3, a continuative – "Ah" – is found only in TT2, and is used to initiate a statement for Silly Young to start chanting and asking for money.

Example 3.3 (adapted from Lao 1999: 236–237, 2004: 194–195)

ST: 明天 好,
PY: míng tiān hǎo
IG: tomorrow good
BT: Tomorrow is good,
TT1: Tomorrow's fine,
TT2: **Ah,** tomorrow'll be beautiful,

The translator of TT2 prefers to add such continuatives as textual Themes, compared to the translator of TT1. As shown in Example 3.4, the continuative "Now" is added in TT2 for Silly Young to draw the attention of the little girl – his addressee – even though no equivalent continuative is used in the ST. In TT1, we only find the interpersonal Theme "Sweet young lady" used to address the little girl.

Example 3.4 (adapted from Lao 1999: 240–241, 2004: 196–197)

ST: 小 姑娘， 别 这样，
PY: xiǎo gū niang, bié zhè yàng,
IG: little girl NEG this
BT: Little girl, don't be like this.
TT1: <u>Sweet young lady, dry</u> your eyes;
TT2: **Now, little girl, don't be** so forlorn,

One instance of conjunctive Adjunct is found in TT2, which is used to recreate the text cohesively. Semantically, the conjunctive Adjunct functions like the conjunction (Halliday & Matthiessen 2014). As shown in Example 3.5, the translator of TT2 adds "after all" to the second half of the sentence, to logico-semantically link the clause to the previous one and to build a parallel structure with the initial part of the line: "With the crowd of well-wishers, I'll now mingle." Also, the two paralleled parts rhyme with each other with the help of "mingle" and "jingle." In this way, the rhymed couplet of the ST is recreated by the translator of TT2.

Example 3.5 (adapted from Lao 1999: 230–231, 2004: 188–189)

ST: [ø:我] 编 点 新 词
PY: wǒ biān diǎn xīn cí
IG: I make up some new words
BT: I make up some new words.
我 也 了不起。
PY: wǒ yě liǎo bù qǐ
IG: I also great
BT: I am also great.
TT1: <u>I</u>'m good at rhymes.
TT2: **After all,** I'm great at making up some jingle!

3.2.2 Analysis of interpersonal Theme in dramatic monologue

For interpersonal Themes, only one interrogative element – "哪位" (PY: nǎ wèi; IG: which) and two Vocatives – "小 姑娘" (PY: xiǎo gū niang; IG: little girl) are found in the ST (see Table 3.3). However, more types of interpersonal Themes are added in the TTs, especially in TT2, such as Finite verbal operators like "would" and "don't," and modal/comment Adjuncts like "never" and "no wonder." The Finite verbal operators are added as a result of typological variations. As there is no Finite in Chinese, translators have to add them as interpersonal Themes in the TTs when translating imperatives with negative polarity or different types of interrogatives from Chinese to English. In Example 3.6, while translating "哪 位" (PY: nǎ wèi; IG: which MEAS) in an elemental interrogative, both translators add "would," which functions as an interpersonal Theme. Also, an additional Vocative – "Old timer there" – is added in TT1.

Table 3.3 Frequency of interpersonal Theme in the
analysis of dramatic monologue

	ST	*TT1*	*TT2*
Vocative	2	3	3
Finite verbal operator	0	2	4
interrogative element	1	0	0
modal/comment Adjunct	0	0	2
Total	3	5	9

Example 3.6 (adapted from Lao 1999: 232–232, 2004: 190–191)

ST: 哪 位 爷, 愿意 听,
PY: nǎ wèi yé, yuàn yì tīng,
IG: which MEAS gentleman want to hear
BT: Which gentleman want to hear?
TT1: <u>Old timer there,</u> **would** <u>you</u> like to hear the scene // About Yang Yan-
zhao and Mu Guiying?
TT2: **Would** <u>you</u> like a story to cheer you up // Of heroes and heroines,

For the modal/comment Adjuncts added as interpersonal Themes in TT2, they are
largely a result of the translator's personal choices. As illustrated in Example 3.7,
the translator of TT2 adds "no wonder" to express his own assessment of the
proposition that the empress dowager is angry.

Example 3.7 (adapted from Lao 1999: 232–233, 2004: 190–191)

ST: [ø:这 件 事] 气 得 太后
PY: zhèi jiàn shì qì de tài hòu
IG: this MEAS event enrage VPART empress dowager
BT: This event enraged the empress dowager
[ø:太后] 咬 牙
PY: tài hòu yǎo yá
IG: empress dowager grind tooth
BT: The empress dowager ground her teeth.
[ø:太后] 切 齿
PY: tài hòu qiè chǐ
IG: empress dowager grind tooth
BT: The empress dowager ground her teeth.
TT1: <u>She</u> raged,
<u>she</u> ground her teeth
and [ø:she] cursed.
TT2: **No wonder** <u>the Empress Dowager</u> was enraged.

Vocatives that function as interpersonal Themes are added to the two TTs. These
Vocatives can be borrowed from the Subject in the ST. As seen in Example 3.8,

the translator of TT2 has translated "王掌柜" (PY: wáng zhǎng guì; IG: Manager Wang) – the unmarked topical Theme in the ST as the interpersonal Theme, i.e. "Manager Wang." Since the next several clauses are all addressed to the manager of the teahouse, the interpersonal Theme can in this way mark out the hearer onstage explicitly. The translator of TT1, however, has put the Vocative – "Proprietor Wang" – in Rheme position, and rhymes "Wang" with "wrong" in the previous line of the playscript.

Example 3.8 (adapted from Lao 1999: 232–233, 2004: 190–191)

ST: 王掌柜, 大 发 财'
PY: wáng zhǎng guì, dà fā cái
IG: Manager Wang big make fortune
BT: Manager Wang will make a great fortune.
TT1: You've made your pile, <<if I'm not wrong,>> // Of silver and gold, Proprietor Wang.
TT2: **Manager Wang**, for you these seem profitable times,

3.2.3 *Analysis of topical Theme in dramatic monologue*

Based on the analysis of topical Theme, we find that the two translators have various strategies in translating topical Themes in the ST. For instance, the topical Theme in the ST can be rendered equivalently in the TTs, such as "我" (PY: wǒ; IG: I) and "I." Some minor changes can be made while translating a topical Theme, such as "王掌柜" (PY: wáng zhǎng guì; IG: Manager Wang) in the ST, "our old proprietor" and "old Proprietor Wang" in TT1, and "poor old Wang" in TT2. Also, it is found that in both TTs, especially TT2, the translators have added various additional topical Themes. Some of the Themes are translated from the Rhemes in the ST, some are the combination of several topical Themes in the ST, and some cannot be traced in the ST. Example 3.9 shows how the topical Themes in the ST, i.e. "天" (PY: tiān; IG: heaven) and "地" (PY: dì; IG: earth) are combined into the topical Theme in TT2 – "What in the heavens above or the earth below." However, the topical Theme – "the country" – in TT1 is translated neither from the Theme nor from the Rheme in the ST.

Example 3.9 (adapted from Lao 1999: 240–241, 2004: 196–197)

ST: 天 可怜,
PY: tiān kě lián,
IG: heaven pitiful
BT: The heaven is pitiful.
地 可怜,
PY: dì kě lián,
IG: earth pitiful
BT: The earth is pitiful.
就是 官 老 爷 有 洋 钱。

PY: jiù shì guān lǎo ye yǒu yáng qián
IG: only official master have foreign money
BT: Only the officials have foreign money.
TT1: **The country** too's in a terrible mess,
Though **the Big Shots** roll in foreign cash.
TT2: **What in the heavens above or the earth below**, // Can stop the
officials from having all the dough?

Table 3.4 and Table 3.5 summarize the frequencies of topical Themes and their
realizations. We can see that fewer participants are found in TT1 and TT2. For TT2,
it is because the translator deliberately selects various circumstances as marked topical Themes; thus, a much larger number of marked choices are found in TT2. For
instance, in Example 3.10, the translator of TT2 purposely chooses "Tasty meat
balls" as the marked topical Theme, so as to put "claim" in the culminative position
and to rhyme "claim" with "game" in the previous line, i.e. "Here chess players meet
for their favorite game." Also, we find a rhymed choice in TT1 –
"play" and "pay," with "loses" functioning as the topical Theme and "pay" as Rheme.

Example 3.10 (adapted from Lao 1999: 230–231, 2004: 188–189)

ST: [ø:您] 赌 一 卖 （碟） 干 炸 丸子
PY: nín dǔ yí mài dié gān zhá wán zi
IG: you (HON) bet one MEAS plate dry fried meatball
BT: You bet for a plate of deep fried meatballs.
TT1: and [ø: you] play // For a plate of meatballs – losers pay.
TT2: **Tasty meat balls**, the winners claim.

Table 3.4 Frequency of topical Theme in the analysis of dramatic monologue

	ST	TT1	TT2
participant	147	121	107
process	4	5	5
circumstance	3	8	22
Total	154	134	134

Table 3.5 Frequency of marked and unmarked topical Theme in the analysis of dramatic monologue

	ST	TT1	TT2
marked topical Theme	4	8	28
unmarked topical Theme	150	126	106
Total	154	134	134

In the ST and TT1, a much smaller amount of marked topical Themes (three and eight respectively) are found compared to TT2. The reason for choosing marked topical Themes is to make the two couplets rhyme, or to make the storytelling rhythmic and chantable. In Example 3.11, Lao She puts "这些 事" (PY: zhèi xiē shì; IG: these matter) – the Complement of the clause – as the marked topical Theme in the ST, instead of choosing the unmarked option, i.e. "别 多 说 这些 事" (PY: bié duō shuō zhèi xiē shì; IG: NEG much talk these matter). Together with the next line "说 着 说 着 就 许 掉 脑壳" (PY: shuō zhe shuō zhe jiù xǔ diào nǎo ké; IG: say VPART say VPART VADV perhaps lose head), the couplets sound smooth in this way. Similarly, in TT1, "the less" functions as the marked topical Theme, while "reform" is in culminative position, so as to form a consonance with "harm" in the next line: "The longer you'll keep your head from harm."

Example 3.11 (adapted from Lao 1999: 232–233, 2004: 190–191)

ST: <u>这些 事</u>,   别 多 说,
PY: zhèi xiē shì, bié duō shuō,
IG: these matters NEG much say
BT: Don't say too much about these matters.
TT1: So **the less** you say about reform.
TT2: <u>But I</u>'d better stop.

More marked topical Themes are found in TT2, indicating the translator's concern for performability and the choice at the expression plane of language while translating the rhymed couplets. In most cases, the translator of TT2 tends to adopt this translation strategy because of the rhyming pattern. As shown in Example 3.12, "For you" functions as the marked topical Theme in TT2, while "times" is put in culminative position as part of the Rheme, so that "times" can rhyme with "rhymes" in the subsequent line. We can see that the translator of TT2 does not make choices such as "These seem profitable times for you" and "You are rich," as such potential choices are not suitable for the rhyming pattern. The translator of TT1, on the other hand, chooses "You" as the unmarked topical Theme, which is equivalent to "您" (PY: nín; IG: you [HON]) in the ST. Because "You've got money" is in the first part of the line of the verse, i.e. "You've got money, but all I own // Is a hungry ballad-monger's tongue," the translator does not have to rhyme with "money."

Example 3.12 (adapted from Lao 1999: 232–233, 2004: 192–193)

ST: 您 有 钱,
PY: nín yǒu qián
IG: you (HON) have money
BT: You have money,
TT1: <u>You</u>'ve got money,
TT2: <u>Manager Wang</u>, **for you** these seem profitable times,

A smaller number of participants are found in TT1 compared to the ST. It is because TT1 tends to be epitomized while translating some clauses that are similar in structure. Example 3.13 shows how four clauses in the ST are rendered as one clause in TT1, with the paralleled clauses in the ST being summarized and condensed.

Example 3.13 (adapted from Lao 1999: 228–229, 2004: 188–189)

ST: [ø:大 茶馆] 茶座 多,
PY: dà chá guǎn chá zuò duō,
IG: big teahouse seat many
BT: The big teahouse has many seats,
[ø: 大 茶 馆] 真 热闹,
PY: dà chá guǎn zhēn rè nao,
IG: big teahouse really bustling
BT: the big teahouse is really bustling,
[ø: 大 茶 馆] 也 有 老 来
PY: dà chá guǎn yě yǒu lǎo lái
IG: big teahouse also have old MOD
BT: the big teahouse also has old people
[ø: 大 茶 馆] 也 有 少;
PY: dà chá guǎn yě yǒu shào;
IG: big teahouse also have young
BT: the big teahouse also has young people
TT1: There's lots of seats and lots of fun, // And lots of folk both old and young;
TT2: Trade is brisk,
lots of tea [ø: are] sold,
Everyone [ø: is] welcome, young and old.

3.3 Theme shift in dramatic monologue

As previously discussed, Matthiessen (2014b) has examined translation shifts by intersecting the metafunctions of the source language with those of the target language. Following this approach, various types of metafunctional translation shifts are identified (see Figure 1.5). When Theme shifts take place, the translators' choices will remain within the textual metafunction, and the textual choices in the TTs will diverge from those in the ST.

Based on the comparison of the Theme choices in the ST and the two TTs, we observe different kinds of Theme shift. In Table 3.6, we categorize these shifts and provide their frequencies. For Theme addition and omission, we point out the more delicate categories according to the elements added, such as addition of conjunction, addition of continuative, and omission of participant. For Theme substitution, no delicate categories are described. Quantitatively, we find a similar number of Theme shifts in TT1 and TT2 (173 and 183 respectively), even though many different Theme choices are found between the two TTs and different translation

Table 3.6 Different types of Theme shift in the analysis of dramatic monologue

Types of Theme shift		*freq. in TT1*	*freq. in TT2*
Theme addition	conjunction	48	37
	continuative	1	3
	continuative Adjunct	0	1
	modal/comment Adjunct	0	2
	Finite verbal operator	2	4
	Vocative	1	1
	participant	8	14
Theme omission	conjunction	1	1
	interrogative element	1	1
	participant	31	32
Theme substitution		78	87
Total		173	183

strategies are adopted by both translators, as demonstrated in previous studies (e.g. Ren 2008). For both TTs, Theme substitution has the largest frequency (78 and 87), while the second most frequent type is Theme addition (60 and 62). In the following subsections, we will introduce the categories of Theme shifts, illustrating them and discussing their frequencies in both TTs.

3.3.1   *Theme addition in dramatic monologue*

Among the different types of Theme addition, the addition of conjunctions is the most frequently found – this reveals the typological differences between Chinese and English and coincides with findings in other studies (see e.g. Ma 2018). The added conjunctions are mostly "and," "or," "but," "although," "so," "when," "while," "for," "nor," and "till," which play cohesive roles in linking clauses with the previous discourse. In Example 3.14, both translators add conjunctions that function as textual Themes to explicitly mark out the logico-semantic relations, including "So" in TT1 and "But" and "and" in TT2.

Example 3.14 (adapted from Lao 1999: 232–233, 2004: 190–191)

ST: 这些 事, 别 多 说
PY: zhèi xiē shì, bié duō shuō
IG: these matters NEG much say
BT: Don't say too much about these matters.
[ø: 您] 说 着
PY: nín shuō zhe
IG: you (HON) say VPART
BT: you say

[ø: 您] 说 着
PY: nín shuō zhe
IG: you (HON) say VPART
BT: you say
[ø: 您] 就 许 掉 脑 壳。
PY: nín jiù xǔ diào nǎo ké
IG: you (HON) VADV may drop head
BT: You may be beheaded.
TT1: <u>So the less</u> you say about reform.
<u>The longer</u> you'll keep your head from harm.
TT2: **But I**'d better stop
and hold myself in check,

Most added conjunctions change the textual transitions from implicit in the ST to explicit in the TTs, thus leading to translation shift from textual to logical meta-function (Matthiessen 2014b). As shown in Example 3.15 (Table 3.7), no textual Theme is found in the ST, while several of them are found in the TTs, including "But" in TT1 and "But," "For," and "nor" in TT2. In the ST, all textual transitions are implicit; hence, readers or the audience would have to make their own inference. However, in both TTs, the transitions, such as those of elaboration (=) and enhancement (×), are made explicit via the addition of cohesive conjunctions. One can note that the Chinese monologue is written in the form of doggerel, so that textual connectors are seldom used. As previously discussed, according to the couplet style of the storytelling, the numbers of the Chinese characters in two adjacent lines are normally the same. Conjunctions in Chinese, such as "然后" (PY: rán hòu; IG: and), "可是" (PY: kě shì; IG: but), "因为" (PY: yīn wéi; IG:

Table 3.7 Example 3.15

Tactic structure	ST	Tactic structure	TT1	Tactic structure	TT2
1α	[ø: 他] 动 脑筋, PY: tā dòng nǎo jīn, IG: he use brain BT: He uses his brain,	1	**But** all his effort is in vain;	α	**But** all his efforts, alas, are looking pretty thin,
1=β	[ø: 他] 白 费 力, PY: tā bái fèi lì, IG: he NEG waste strength BT: He wastes his strength,	=2	There are certain things you can't attain.	×β α	**For** with heads he lost,
×2	胳膊 拧 不 过 大腿 去。 PY: gē bo nǐng bú guò dà tuǐ qù IG: arm wring NEG CV thigh PV BT: An arm cannot compete with a leg.			×β+β	**nor** with tails did win.

Source: Adapted from Lao (1999: 234–235, 2004: 192–193)

because) will not only be regarded as redundant but will also destroy the rhythmic pattern in Chinese.

In terms of the frequency of the conjunctions as textual Themes, 48 and 37 of them are added in the TTs. The quantitative difference reveals the two translators' preference for such choices. Compared with the translator of TT2, the translator of TT1 tends to add more conjunctions as textual Themes. As shown in Example 3.16, even though no conjunction functions as a textual Theme in the ST, two of them, i.e. "and" and "when," are added in TT1. The use of "And" links the first clause in TT1 to the previous one – "The Emperor's prestige is daily less" by way of extension (+), while "when" connects the two clauses in the example by way of enhancement (×).

Example 3.16 (adapted from Lao 1999: 230–231, 2004: 190–191)

ST: 文 武 官, 有 一 宝,
PY: wén wǔ guān, yǒu yì bǎo,
IG: civil military officer have one trick
BT: Civil and military officers have one trick,

[ø: 文 武 官] 见 着 洋人
PY: wén wǔ guān jiàn zhao yáng rén
IG: civil military officer see VPART foreigner
BT: civil and military officers see a foreigner

[ø: 文 武 官] 赶快 跑。
PY: wén wǔ guān gǎn kuài pǎo
IG: civil military officer quickly run
BT: civil and military officers quickly run.

TT1: **And** our Ministers, military and civil // Run
when they see a foreign devil.

TT2: Mandarins and generals have one common trick,
Faced by foreign armies,
they turn tail double quick.

In general, the frequencies of the added textual Themes coincide with the amount of conjunctions functioning as textual Themes in the TTs (see Table 3.2). Examples of continuative addition can be found in Examples 3.3 and 3.4, while Example 3.5 illustrates the one occurrence of the addition of a conjunctive Adjunct in TT2.

In terms of the addition of interpersonal Theme, the additions of Finite verbal operators are attributed to the typological differences between Chinese and English. As previously stated, no Finite is described in the interpersonal grammar of Chinese, whereas for declaratives and interrogatives in English, the syntagmatic order of Subject and Finite plays a crucial role in determining the mood types of the clauses. When translating imperatives with negative polarity or interrogatives from Chinese to English, in which Finites function as interpersonal Themes, translators have to add the Finite verbal operators to the TTs, although such elements are not found in Chinese (see Example 3.6). The frequency of additions of this type is low, as the mood types of most clauses in dramatic monologue (both in the ST and the TTs) are declaratives.

In contrast, some additions, such as those of continuative (see Example 3.3), modal/comment Adjunct (see Example 3.7) and Vocative (Example 3.6) are largely the translators' personal preference. Example 3.17 shows how a modal/comment Adjunct is added as an interpersonal Theme in TT2. The lexical choice of "莫" (PY: mò; IG: NEG), which means "不要" (PY: bú yào; IG: NEG), reveals the negative polarity in the ST. In TT2, we find the addition of modality of usuality realized by "Never," which functions as interpersonal Theme and differs from the interpersonal meaning in the ST.

Example 3.17 (adapted from Lao 1999: 230–231, 2004: 190–191)

ST: 莫 谈 国 事
PY: mò tán guó shì
IG: NEG discuss state affair
BT: Don't discuss state affairs.
您 得 老 记着。
PY: nín děi lǎo jì zhe
IG: you (HON) have to always remember
BT: You have to always remember.
TT1: If you'd keep your pate,
You'd better not talk about affairs of state.
TT2: **Never**, <<if you please,>> discuss affairs of state.

The additions of participants as topical Themes are associated with the additions of clauses. Some of these clauses have no equivalents in the ST (see Example 3.18), and some are repetitive, forming extensive relations in the clause complexes (see Example 3.19). In Example 3.18, we find an additional clause in TT1 – "or I'm a liar" – with "or" and "I" functioning as the added textual and topical Themes respectively. Moreover, the topical Theme in the ST is substituted by "There" in TT1 and "For your grand opening" in TT2. We should also note that "八 蜡 庙" (PY: bā là miào; IG: eight deity temple) is the name of a Peking opera, which tells the story of how heroes and an upright official punish a local tyrant. The lexical choice of "庙" (PY: miào; IG: temple) here rhymes with "炮" (PY: pào; IG: cannon) in the previous clause "他 开 炮" (PY: tā kāi pào; IG: he fire cannon).

Example 3.18 (adapted from Lao 1999: 236–237, 2004: 194–195)

ST: 明天 准 唱 《八 蜡 庙》
PY: míng tiān zhǔn chàng bā là miào
IG: tomorrow certainly perform eight deity temple
BT: Tomorrow there will certainly be performance of *Eight Deity Temple*
TT1: There'll be trouble tomorrow
or I'm a liar.
TT2: For your grand opening they may spoil the show.

In terms of the frequency of topical Theme addition, the occurrence in TT2 is higher than that of TT1. Example 3.19 shows how two clauses with similar meanings are added in TT2, leading to the addition of topical Themes. For instance, in Example 3.19, two additional clauses – "or hum" and "others sit" – are added in TT2. They help to make this line rhythmic and of the same length with the other lines. The translator of TT1, on the other hand, chooses to translate in a more equivalent way, and no extra clause is added.

Example 3.19 (adapted from Lao 1999: 228–229, 2004: 188–189)

ST: 有的 说，
PY: yǒu de shuō,
IG: some talk
BT: Some talk.
有的 唱，
PY: yǒu de chàng,
IG: some sing
BT: Some sing.
TT1: Some of them talk,
and some of them sing –
TT2: Some sing,
or [ø: some] hum,
others sit
and [ø: others] chat,

3.3.2 Theme omission in dramatic monologue

When Theme omission takes place, the Theme in the ST is no longer translated equivalently into the TTs; instead, it is left out untranslated. According to our analysis, the omitted Theme can be textual, interpersonal, and topical, and the frequencies of Theme omission in both TTs are similar.

In terms of textual Theme omission, we find that the one conjunction that functions as a textual Theme in the ST, i.e. "自从" (PY: zì cóng; IG: since), is omitted in both TTs. Both translators choose to render the clauses in the TTs as free ones rather than as bound ones beginning with "since," which have to be used along with free clauses (see Example 3.20). In TT1, we also note that the translator adds "Old Beijing, old China's pride," which has no equivalent in the ST, so as to rhyme "pride" with "occupied." In TT2, there is the possibility of putting the prepositional phrase – "For eight years" – at the beginning of the clause to function as the marked topical Theme, which is, in fact, found at the end in the culminative position. This is because the translator tries to rhyme "years" with "tears" in the next clause – "Those were the days of blood and tears."

Example 3.20 (adapted from Lao 1999: 238–239, 2004: 194–195)

ST: 自从 那, 日本 兵, 八 年 占据 老 北京。
PY: zì cóng nà, rì běn bīng, bā nián zhàn jù lǎo běi jīng
IG: since that Japanese soldier eight year occupy old Beijing
BT: since the Japanese soldier occupied old Beijing for eight years
TT1: <u>Eight years</u> the Japanese occupied // Old Beijing, old China's pride.
TT2: <u>The Japs</u> held old Beijing for eight long years.

For omission of interpersonal Theme, one omission of interrogative element is found in both TTs. As illustrated in Example 3.21, the mood type of the first clause in the ST is analyzed as an elemental interrogative, and "哪 位 爷" (PY: nǎ wèi yé; IG: which MEAS gentleman) functions as both the interpersonal Theme and unmarked topical Theme. In both TTs, this interpersonal Theme is omitted, as both translators have not rendered the elemental interrogative as wh- interrogative, which is the equivalent mood type in English.

Example 3.21 (adapted from Lao 1999: 232–233, 2004: 190–191)

ST: 哪 位 爷, 愿意 听,
PY: nǎ wèi yé, yuàn yì tīng,
IG: which MEAS gentleman want to hear
BT: Which gentleman wants to hear?
《 辕门 斩 子 》 来 了 穆桂英。
PY: yuán mén zhǎn zǐ lái le mù guì yīng
IG: gate behead son come ASP Mu Guiying
BT: There comes Mu Guiying in *Son to Be Killed at the Gate*.
TT1: <u>Old timer there, would you</u> like to hear the scene // About Yang Yanzhao and Mu Guiying?
TT2: <u>Would you</u> like a story to cheer you up // Of heroes and heroines, while <u>you</u> enjoy your cup?

Omissions of topical Theme from the ST are of similar frequencies in the two TTs, and the omitted topical Themes are all realized by participants. In the ST, similar ideas are frequently repeated in various contiguous clauses, whereas in the TTs, such information may not necessarily be repeated. Therefore, many Themes are omitted when two or more clauses in the ST are combined into one clause in the TTs (see also Example 3.13). Example 3.22 shows how Themes, especially topical Themes, are omitted when clauses with similar meaning in the ST are combined in the TTs. In TT1, the three clauses in the ST are reduced to one clause. Two identical topical Themes, i.e. "人" (PY: rén; IG: man), are omitted, while one is replaced by "an old man's back," which is translated from part of the Rheme in the second clause of the ST. In TT2, one topical Theme in the ST is omitted, while one is replaced with "their backs."

Example 3.22 (adapted from Lao 1999: 238–239, 2004: 194–195)

ST: 人 老
PY: rén lǎo
IG: man old
BT: Man is old.
[ø: 人] 毛 腰
PY: rén máo yāo
IG: man bend back
BT: Man bends his back.
[ø: 人] 把 头 低
PY: rén bǎ tóu dī
IG: man CV head lower
BT: Man lowers his head.
TT1: <u>An old man's back</u> is bent with care.
TT2: <u>When men</u> are old,
<u>their backs</u> are bent.

Some omissions of participants that function as topical Themes are due to clause omission. These shifts are often seen in TT2. As shown in Example 3.23, both translators have left the second clause in the ST untranslated, leading to the omissions of "我" (PY: wǒ; IG: I), which functions as the topical Theme in the ST. In addition, Theme substitutions take place when the topical Theme in the first clause in the ST – "人人" (PY: rén; IG: everybody) – is translated as "The people" and "Those" in both TTs respectively.

Example 3.23 (adapted from Lao 1999: 238–239, 2004: 194–195)

ST: 人人 苦,
PY: rén rén kǔ,
IG: everybody painful
BT: Everybody was painful,
[ø: 我] 没法 提,
PY: wǒ méi fǎ tí,
IG: I cannot mention
BT: I cannot mention
TT1: <u>The people</u> suffered without relief,
TT2: <u>Those</u> were the days of blood and tears.

3.3.3 *Theme substitution in dramatic monologue*

When Theme substitution takes place, the Theme in the ST is substituted by an inequivalent element in the TTs, which may be translated from the Rheme in the ST or from nowhere. This kind of shift is the most frequently found Theme shift in our analysis (see Table 3.6). The frequency in TT2 is relatively higher than that in TT1, and it indicates the free strategy of translation adopted by the translator. As shown in Example 3.24, the two translators choose to substitute "人" (PY: rén; IG: man) – the topical Theme in the ST with "a lot of people" and "Our pigtails" respectively, leading to Theme substitutions.

Example 3.24 (adapted from Lao 1999: 234–235, 2004: 192–193)

ST: [ø: 人] 剪 了 小 辫
PY: rén jiǎn le xiǎo biàn
IG: man cut ASP little pigtail
BT: Men cut the little pigtails
TT1: <u>But a lot of people</u> still wear queues.
TT2: <u>Our pigtails</u> were cut off,

When Theme substitution takes place, the Theme in the ST may be replaced by its synonym or a related word/phrase in the TTs. In Example 3.25, we find "茶馆" (PY: chá guǎn; IG: teahouse) in the ST substituted by "His place" in TT2 – a different lexical choice that still refers to the teahouse. By the same token, we often find "王掌柜" (PY: wáng zhǎng guì; IG: Manager Wang) – the topical Theme in several clauses in the ST – translated as "our old Proprietor" in TT1 and "Poor old Wang" in TT2.

Example 3.25 (adapted from Lao 1999: 236–237, 2004: 192–193)

ST: 茶馆 好像 大学堂,
PY: chá guǎn hǎo xiàng dà xué táng,
IG: teahouse be like college
BT: Teahouse is like a college.
TT1: <u>[ø: Manager Wang]</u> Has turned his shop into a seat of learning.
TT2: <u>His place</u> has the air of a boarding school.

The translators may choose to add more experiential meaning to the topical Theme in the ST. For instance, in Example 3.26, the translator of TT2 adds "victories" to "the Eighth Route Army," even though no equivalent of "victories," such as "胜利" (PY: shèng lì), is found in the topical Theme in the ST – "好 八路" (PY: hǎo bā lù; IG: good Eight Route Army).

Example 3.26 (adapted from Lao 1999: 238–239, 2004: 194–195)

ST: 好 八路, 得 人 心
PY: hǎo bā lù, dé rén xīn
IG: good Eighth Route Army win people heart
BT: The good Eighth Route Army won people's heart
TT1: <u>But the Eighth Route Army</u> won their heads
TT2: <u>The Eighth Route Army's victories,</u> [ø: are] the only source of mirth.

One of the motivations for the two translators to substitute the topical Theme in the ST with an inequivalent one is the concern of rhyme in the translation. In TT2, we find that the translator chooses to thematize the Rhemes in the ST by translating them as marked topical Themes. According to Example 3.27, in the ST, the character "京" (PY: jīng; IG: Beijing) in "北京" (PY: běi jīng; IG: Beijing) rhymes with "兵" (PY: bīng; IG: soldier) in the next line of the verse. Both translators have tried to recreate the rhyme scheme when translating the ST into English. In TT1, "Beijing" rhymes with "everything"; while in TT2, the circumstance – "to Old Beijing" – is translated as the Theme in the clause, with "the KMT" being put at the end in culminative position, so as to rhyme "KMT" with "be." Therefore, to ensure that the TTs are chantable, the translator of TT2 deliberately chooses lexical choices that rhyme with each other and puts them at the end of the line, despite the various changes made to the Theme and Rheme position. In other words, the shifts here at the lexicogrammar stratum are to maintain the equivalence elsewhere on the expression plane and at the phonology stratum (cf. Halliday 2009, 2010).

Example 3.27 (adapted from Lao 1999: 238–239, 2004: 196–197)

ST: 国民党，进 北京，
PY: guó mín dǎng, jìn běi jīng,
IG: Kuomintang enter Beijing
BT: Kuomintang enters Beijing.
TT1: <u>Now</u> the Kuomintang are in Beijing,
TT2: <u>Then to Old Beijing</u> came the KMT!

Theme substitution may be related to shift of mood type. As shown in Example 3.28, the imperative: jussive in the first clause of the ST is translated as a declarative in both TTs. Thus, the lexical choice of "甭" (PY: béng; IG: do NEG), realized by a process, is substituted by participants, namely "I" in TT1 and "it" in TT2.

Example 3.28 (adapted from Lao 1999: 238–239, 2004: 194–195)

ST: 甭 说 (mood type: imperative: jussive)
PY: béng shuō
IG: do say
BT: Don't say
我， 混 不 了 (mood type: declarative)
PY: wǒ, hùn bù liǎo
IG: I drift along NEG ASP
BT: I did not drift along
TT1: <u>I</u>'m finding it hard (mood type: declarative)
[ø: I] to get along; (mood type: bound)
TT2: [ø: it is] Needless to say, (mood type: declarative)
<u>I</u>'m done for altogether. (mood type: bound)

Alternatively, when a declarative in the ST is translated as an imperative in the TTs, a shift in Theme substitution is likely to be involved. In Example 3.29, "茶馆" (PY: chá guǎn; IG: teahouse), the topical Theme in the ST, is changed to "pray" in TT2, which is realized by a process and signals the mood choice of imperative.

Example 3.29 (adapted from Lao 1999: 236–237, 2004: 192–193)

ST: [ø: 茶馆] 就 怕 呀, 兵 野蛮 (mood type: declarative)
PY: chá guǎn jiù pà ya, bīng yě mán
IG: teahouse VADV be afraid of MOD soldier brutish
BT: The teahouse is afraid of brutish soldiers,
TT1: <u>Then the soldiers</u> come, (mood type: declarative)
TT2: <u>But pray</u> to Heaven (mood type: imperative: jussive)
<u>no brutish soldiers</u> come, (mood type: bound)

Some Theme substitutions reflect the differences between English and Chinese. When translating existential clauses in Mandarin Chinese (or relational: existential according to Halliday & McDonald 2004: 364–366), translators may replace the circumstance that functions as the unmarked topical Theme in the ST with "there" in the TTs. This typological difference is illustrated in Example 3.30, where the translator of TT1 substitutes the original Theme "大 茶馆" (PY: dà chá guǎn; IG: big teahouse) with "there." The translator of TT2, on the other hand, makes another choice by changing the existential process to another process type, i.e. relational: identifying.

Example 3.30 (adapted from Lao 1999: 230–231, 2004: 188–189)

ST: [ø: 大 茶馆] 有 提 笼
PY: dà chá guǎn yǒu tí lóng
IG: big teahouse have carry cage
BT: Big teahouse has people carrying bird cages.
[ø: 大 茶馆] 有 架 鸟
PY: dà chá guǎn yǒu jià niǎo
IG: big teahouse have carry bird
BT: Big teahouse has people carrying birds.
TT1: <u>There</u>'s birds,
TT2: <u>This</u> is where bird fanciers meet,

3.4 Summary

This chapter discussed the textual choices made in the ST and the two TTs of the dramatic monologue of *Teahouse*. We have reported the findings of our quantitative analysis of Theme and pointed out some different choices made by the two translators. Also, we have introduced the various categories of Theme shift – the translation shifts remaining within the textual metafunction (Matthiessen 2014b), including Theme addition, Theme omission, and Theme substitution. Additionally, some delicate types of shifts were discussed and exemplified. We have related the translators' concern for performability to the choices they make. As revealed in various examples used in this chapter, the rhymed pattern of the dramatic mono-logue has largely influenced the textual choices made by the two translators. In order to rhyme every two lines and to make the storytelling rhythmic, a free way of translation is adopted, and the textual choices are thus not always translated by their closest English equivalents.

In this chapter, the Chinese rhythmic storytelling has for one of the first times been analyzed in light of SFL. As a unique art form, rhythmic storytelling was seldom studied from a linguistic perspective (cf. Shih 2012). The findings revealed some unique linguistic features in the Chinese ST and its English TTs and could help us to gain a better understanding of this particular register. In various previous studies, the dramatic monologue in *Teahouse* was not considered in the analysis (e.g. Ren 2008), as attention was primarily given to dramatic dialogue, which plays a more significant role in the play and constitutes the largest part of the play. Therefore, the analysis in this chapter has shed more light on the comparative studies of *Teahouse* and its different English translations.

Some typological similarities and differences between English and Chinese can be observed based on the lexicogrammatical analysis of Theme.

First, the basic choices in the system of THEME are similar in English and Chi-nese. Choices of textual Theme and interpersonal Theme are optional in major clauses, and choices of topical Theme are compulsory. For instance, all the major clauses we analyzed have a topical Theme, such as "大 茶馆" (PY: dà chá guǎn; IG: big teahouse), "There" and "Trade" in Example 3.13, while no textual and interpersonal Theme is found in these clauses.

Second, the topical Theme in the Chinese ST has the potential to be omitted. These omitted topical Themes can be added back in the analysis, such as "这 件 事" (PY: zhèi jiàn shì; IG: this MEAS event) in Example 3.7. In the English TTs, the omission of topical Theme is also possible, for instance, in "And fill the place with cultured talk," the omitted topical Theme is "college students," which is added back in our analysis.

Third, in both languages, the typical order of Theme is textual ^ interpersonal ^ topical. Though textual and interpersonal Themes are rarely found in the Chinese ST, they are always before the topical Theme. For instance, in "自从 那 日本 兵, 八 年 占据 老 北京。" (PY: zì cóng nà rì běn bīng, bā nián zhàn jù lǎo běi jīng; IG: since that Japanese soldier, eight year occupy old Beijing), the textual Theme "自从" (PY: zì cóng; IG: since) is found before the topical Theme "那 日本 兵" (PY: nà rì běn bīng; IG: that Japanese soldier). In "小 姑娘， 别 这样，" (PY: xiǎo gū niang bié zhè yàng; IG: little girl NEG this), the interpersonal Theme realized by the Vocative "小 姑娘" (PY: xiǎo gū niang; IG: little girl) precedes the topical Theme "别" (PY: bié; IG: do NEG). Similar examples are also found in the English TTs, as in "Now, little girl, don't be so forlorn" from TT2, the textual Theme "Now" realized by a continuative, the interpersonal Themes – "little girl" and "don't" – realized by a Vocative and a Finite verbal operator respectively precede the topical Theme "be" realized by a process.

Fourth, unlike English, there is no system of FINITE in Chinese. Therefore, in clauses of imperative and polar interrogative mood, there is no interpersonal Theme realized by a Finite verbal operator in Chinese. For example, in an imperative like "这些 事, 别 多 说" (PY: zhè xiē shì bié duō shuō; IG: these matter NEG much say), there is no Finite, and "这些 事" (PY: zhè xiē shì; IG: these matter) functions as the topical Theme. In the English TTs, Finites can function as interpersonal Themes in yes/no interrogatives and imperatives, such as "Would" in "Would you like a story to cheer you up" and "Don't" in "Don't be hard on poor old me."

Fifth, in the English TTs, circumstances that function as topical Themes are analyzed as marked choices, such as "into the teahouse" in "into the teahouse I go." However, in the Chinese ST, circumstances in clauses whose process types are analyzed as existential or relational: existential are considered as the unmarked topical Themes (cf. Halliday & McDonald 2004). For instance, in "[ø:朝 中] 还 有 那 康有为 和 梁启超" (PY: cháo zhōng hái yǒu nà kāng yǒu wéi hé liáng qǐ chāo; IG: court in also exist that Kang Youwei and Liang Qichao), the circumstance – "朝 中" (PY: cháo zhōng; IG: court in) is here considered as the unmarked topical Theme.

When making choices textually, translators have to choose to interpret the messages and the sequences of messages in the English source text. They also choose to re-present the textual meanings among the options in English (Matthiessen 2014b). Based on the lexicogrammatical analysis of Theme, we can summarize some of their trade-offs as follows.

First, the translators need to add a large number of textual Themes, based on their interpretation of the ST, to recreate the flow of information in the ST and to reproduce a cohesive TT in English. Most of these textual Themes are realized by conjunctions such as "and" and "but" in the TTs. Second, when choosing certain mood types in the English system of MOOD, translators have to be aware of the systemic differences between the two languages. For instance, interpersonal Themes like "would" have to be added in "Old timer there, would you like to hear the scene // About Yang Yanzhao and Mu Guiying?" from TT1. Third, textual choices are sometimes informed by rhyming pattern and performability, making it necessary for translators to resort to translation strategies like dynamic equivalence, communicative equivalence, or covert translation (see Nida 1964; Nida & Taber 1969; Newmark 1988; House 1997, 2015; cf. Wang & Ma 2016).

Notes

1 Part of Section 3.2 has been published in Wang and Ma (2018), which reports on findings from the textual and logical analysis of the dramatic monologue of *Teahouse*.
2 We have underlined the choices of Theme in the examples to illustrate how Theme is analyzed in the present study.

4 Reconstruing logical meaning in stage direction

This chapter discusses the analysis of stage direction from the perspectives of taxis and logico-semantic type. The stage direction in *Teahouse* functions as the notes added by Lao She to provide information not stated in the dramatic dialogue and monologue (cf. Hartnoll & Found 1996). In the present study, we have selected the stage direction in the beginning paragraphs in the three acts of *Teahouse*. These paragraphs introduce both the stage setting and the major characters to readers who may be directors and actors that require further directions from the playwright or literature enthusiasts that appreciate *Teahouse* as a literary work.

In Section 4.1, we first introduce the concepts to be used in the analysis, i.e. systems of TAXIS and LOGICO-SEMANTIC TYPE. In Section 4.2, we analyze and compare the choices made in the stage direction in terms of taxis and logico-semantic type. Section 4.3 examines the two kinds of metafunctional translation shifts involved in the analysis, namely tactic shift and logico-semantic type shift. The delicate categories of these shifts will also be presented. The analyses in Chapters 2, 3, and 4 offer a revealing account of how the discourse of *Teahouse* is organized to effectively function in its context of situation and context of culture.

4.1 A description of taxis and logico-semantic type in systemic functional terms

The logical metafunction and the experiential metafunction are the two modes of experience construal within the ideational metafunction. Within the logical mode, "our experience is construed serially as chains of phenomena related by logico-semantic relationships" (Matthiessen, Teruya & Lam 2010: 150). The major systems that examine how clauses combine with each other to form a clause complex include TAXIS (degree of interdependency) and LOGICO-SEMANTIC TYPE (see Figure 4.1).

TAXIS deals with "the interdependency relations between grammatical units forming a complex, such as groups forming a group complex or clauses forming a clause complex" (Martin, Matthiessen & Painter 2010: 231). There are two options in the system of TAXIS, i.e. parataxis and hypotaxis. A paratactic relationship means that the two units forming the complex are of equal semantic weight.

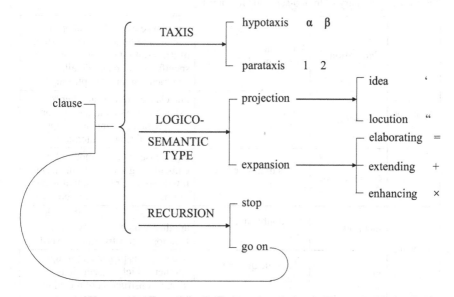

Figure 4.1 The system of clause complexing

Source: Adapted from Halliday & Matthiessen (2014: 438)

If the status is unequal, then it is a hypotactic relationship. Following the SFL conventions, α and other small Greek letters are used to label the elements of hypotactic interdependency structure, while Arabic numerals are used to refer to the elements of paratactic interdependency structure.

There are two logico-semantic types, i.e. expansion and projection. Halliday and Matthiessen (2014: 443) make the following distinctions between the two: "Expansion relates phenomena as being of the same order of experience, while projection relates phenomena of one order of experience (the processes of saying and thinking) to phenomena of a higher order (semiotic phenomena – what people say and think)." Further distinctions of expansion and projection can be made, as shown in Table 4.1.

Example 4.1 (see Table 4.2) illustrates how clause complexes are analyzed in this book. There are three clause simplexes in this clause complex, and the internal nesting can be presented as follows: $1 \wedge +2 \, (\alpha \wedge \times\beta)$. In this example, the first clause simplex and the two remaining ones are paratactically linked by an adversative relation (+), marked by the use of "but," and the last two clauses are hypotactically related by the enhancing relation of purpose (×). The logico-semantic relationship in this clause complex can be visualized with the help of Rhetorical Structure Theory (RST), which is used to represent the rhetorical organization of a text (e.g. Mann, Matthiessen & Thompson 1992), as shown in Figure 4.2.

According to existing systemic functional descriptions of Chinese (e.g. Li 2007), when combining clause simplexes to form a clause complex, the clauses

Table 4.1 A summary of logico-semantic relationships

expansion	elaboration	= ("equals") "i.e., e.g., viz."	one clause expands another by elaborating on it (or some portion of it): restating in other words, specifying in greater detail, commenting, or exemplifying
	extension	+ ("is added to") "and, or"	one clause expands another by extending beyond it: adding some new element, giving an exception to it, or offering an alternative
	enhancement	× ("is multiplied by") "so, yet, then"	one clause expands another by embellishing around it: qualifying it with some circumstantial feature of time, place, cause, or condition
Projection	locution	" " (double quotes) "says"	one clause is projected through another, which presents it as a locution, a construction of wording
	idea	' ' (single quotes) "thinks"	one clause is projected through another, which presents it as an idea, a construction of meaning

Source: Adapted from Halliday & Matthiessen (2014: 444)

Table 4.2 Example 4.1

1	Gang fights were common in those days,
+2 α	but fortunately there were always friends around
+2 ×β	to calm things down.

Source: Adapted from Lao (1999: 3)

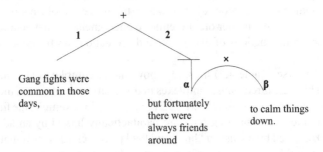

Figure 4.2 The logico-semantic relations in Example 4.1

will enter into the two simultaneous systems of TAXIS and LOGICO-SEMANTIC TYPE. Thus, a clause complex in Chinese can also be analyzed from these two perspectives. In Example 4.2 (see Table 4.3), the relation between the first clause and the remaining two is paratactic elaboration (=), with the final two clauses elaborating

Table 4.3 Example 4.2

1	茶座 也 大 加 改良：
	PY: *chá zuò yě dà jiā gǎi liáng*
	IG: seat also largely CV reform
	BT: *Seats are also largely reformed:*
=2 1	一律 是 小 桌 与 藤 椅，
	PY: yí lǜ shì xiǎo zhuō yǔ téng yǐ
	IG: all be small table and cane chair
	BT: all are small tables and cane chairs.
=2 +2	桌 上 铺 着 浅 绿 桌布。
	PY: zhuō shàng pū zhe qiǎn lǜ zhuō bù
	IG: table on spread light green table cloth
	BT: On the tables there spread light green table cloths.

Source: Adapted from Lao (1999: 58)

on how the reform is carried out. The relationship between the last two clauses is identified as paratactic extension (+), as the third clause is an addition to the preceding one.

4.2 Analysis of taxis and logico-semantic type in stage direction

In Table 4.4, we quantify the number of clause simplexes in one clause complex in the ST and the TTs. In most cases, one clause complex is composed of one to five clause simplexes. For the ST, the preferred choices are two and three clause simplexes, while those of the TTs are one and two clause simplexes. As shown in Example 4.3, one clause complex composed by two clauses is translated as one clause simplex in both TTs (see Table 4.5). In this way, the logico-sematic relation of extension (+) in the ST is omitted in the TTs.

Example 4.4 illustrates how logico-semantic relationship between the ST and the TTs varies (see Table 4.6). The clause complex in the ST consists of the largest number of clause simplexes. However, when translating the final four clause simplexes in the ST, the two translators have reconstrued them as another clause complex in the TTs.

Based on the analysis of taxis, some quantitative differences are observed (see Figure 4.3). Between parataxis and hypotaxis, parataxis is the preferred choice in the ST, while hypotaxis is preferred in TT2. For TT1, the choice of parataxis and hypotaxis is similar in frequency (25 versus 23).

Example 4.5 shows how the choice of taxis varies between the ST and the two TTs (see Table 4.7). A succession of paratactic extending relations is found in the clause complex in the ST to describe the appearance of Tang the Oracle. In the TTs, the paratactic relations are changed to hypotactic, with the use of several non-Finite clauses such as "wearing a very long and very filthy cotton gown" in TT1 and "some scraps of paper tucked into his hat near the temples" in TT2. Moreover, as a result of choosing hypotaxis frequently, the occurrence of hypotaxis in both TTs is higher than that in the ST (see Figure 4.3).

Table 4.4 Number of clause simplexes in one clause complex in the analysis of stage direction

	1 clause	2 clauses	3 clauses	4 clauses	5 clauses	6 clauses	7 clauses	8 clauses
ST	13	15	14	4	3	0	0	1
TT1	21	17	9	4	1	1	0	0
TT2	25	20	4	3	4	0	0	0

Table 4.5 Example 4.3

Tactic structure	ST	Tactic structure	TT1	Tactic structure	TT2
1	总之，这是当日非常重要的地方, PY: zǒng zhī, zhè shì dāng rì fēi cháng zhòng yào de dì fang, IG: in sum this be that time very important place BT: In sum, this is a very import place at that time.	–	In sum, the teahouse was an important institution of those times, a place [[[where people came to transact business, ‖ or simply to while away the time]]].	–	In short, the teahouse was a most important institution, a place [[[where people could come for business ‖ or just to while away the time]]].
+2	有事无事都可以来坐半天。 PY: yǒu shì wú shì dōu kě yǐ lái zuò bàn tiān IG: have business NEG business all can come sit half day BT: People have or have no business can all come in to sit for some time.				

Source: Adapted from Lao (1999: 2–3, 2004: 12–13)

Table 4.6 Example 4.4

Tactic structure	ST	Tactic structure	TT1	Tactic structure	TT2
1 α	那年月，时常有打群架的, PY: nà nián yuè, shí cháng yǒu dǎ qún jià de, IG: those time, often have gang fight SUB BT: In those days, there were often gang fights,	1	In those days there would often be quarrels between gangs	1	Gang fights were common in those days,

Tactic structure	ST	Tactic structure	TT1	Tactic structure	TT2
1 +β	但是 总会 有 朋友 PY: dàn shì zǒng huì yǒu péng you IG: but always have friends BT: but there were always friends	+2 α	but there were always friends about	+2 α	but fortunately there were always friends around
1 +γ	出头 PY: chū tóu IG: appear BT: appear	+2 ×β	to calm things down	+2 ×β	to calm things down.
1 +δ	给 双方 调解； PY: gěi shuāng fāng tiáo jiě; IG: CV both sides mediate BT: mediate for both sides;	1 1	The two sides would crowd around these mediators [[who would reason first with one side then the other]]	1 α α	Between 30 to 50 toughs from both sides, <<reconciled through the good offices of a mediator,>> would gather here
=2 α	三五十 口子 打手，经 调人 东说西说， PY: sān wǔ shí kǒu zi dǎ shǒu, jīng tiáo rén dōng shuō xī shuō, IG: thirty to fifty MEAS fighter, after mediator reconciliation BT: thirty to fifty fighters after the mediator's reconciliation,	1 ×2 1	then they would all drink tea	1 α =β	<<reconciled through the good offices of a mediator,>>
=2 ×β α	便 都 喝 碗 茶， PY: biàn dōu hē wǎn chá, IG: then all drink bowl tea BT: then all drink bowls of tea,	1 ×2 +2	and down bowls of noodle, with minced pork,	1 ×β α	to drink tea
=2 ×β +β	吃 碗 烂肉面， PY: chī wǎn làn ròu miàn, IG: eat bowl minced meat noodle BT: eat bowls of minced-meat noodle	=2	hostility transformed to hospitality.	1 ×β +β	and consume bowls of noodles with minced pork,
=2 ×γ	就 可以 化 干戈 为 玉 帛 了。 PY: jiù kě yǐ huà gān gē wéi yù bó le IG: then can transform hostility to friendship ASP BT: then they can transform hostility to friendship.			×2	and peace would once more have been restored in the land.

Source: Adapted from Lao (1999: 2–3, 2004: 10–13)

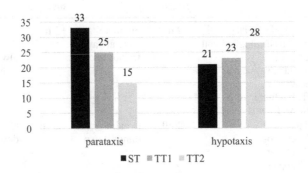

Figure 4.3 Frequency of taxis in the analysis of stage direction

Table 4.7 Example 4.5

Tactic structure	ST	Tactic structure	TT1	Tactic structure	TT2
1	唐铁嘴 踏拉 着鞋， PY: táng tiě zuǐ tā la zhe xié, IG: Tang the Oracle scuff VPART shoe, BT: Tang the Oracle scuffed in his shoes,	α	Soothsayer Tang enters in tattered shoes,	α	Tang the Oracle enters,
+2	身穿一件极长极脏的大布衫， PY: shēn chuān yí jiàn jí cháng jí zāng de dà bù shān, IG: wear one MEAS very long very dirty SUB big gown BT: he wear a very long and dirty big gown,	=β	wearing a very long and very filthy cotton gown,	=β α	his shoes half off his feet,
+3	耳上夹着几张小纸片， PY: ěr shàng jiá zhe jǐ zhāng xiǎo zhǐ piàn, IG: ear on tuck VPART several MEAS little paper scrap BT: he tucks several scraps of paper on his ear,	+γ	some scraps of paper tucked behind one year.	=β +β	and wearing an extremely long and dirty gown,
+4	进来。 PY: jìn lái IG: enter BT: he enters.			=β +γ	some scraps of paper tucked into his hat near the temples.

Source: Adapted from Lao (1999: 8–9, 2004: 14–15)

Table 4.8 Example 4.6

Tactic structure	ST	Tactic structure	TT1	Tactic structure	TT2
1	厨房 挪到 后面 去, PY: chú fáng nuó dào hòu miàn qù, IG: kitchen move back PV BT: The kitchen is moved to the back,	1	The kitchen has been moved out back,	α	The stove has been moved to the back,
+2	专 包 公寓 住客 的 伙食。 PY: zhuān bāo gōng yù zhù kè de huǒ shí IG: specially serve apartment lodger SUB meal BT: specially serves meals for lodgers in the apartment.	+2	and only serves meals for the lodgers.	×β	**for** preparing meals for the lodgers.

Source: Adapted from Lao (1999: 8–9, 2004: 14–15)

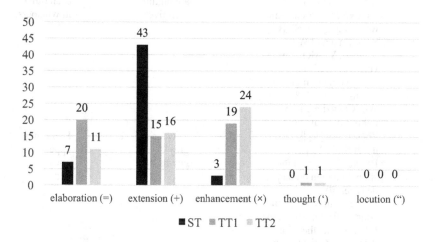

Figure 4.4 Frequency of logico-semantic type in the analysis of stage direction

In addition, the frequency of parataxis in TT2 is the smallest and that of hypotaxis is the largest, compared to the occurrences in the ST and TT1 (see Figure 4.3). As shown in Example 4.6 (see Table 4.8), the paratactic relation is equivalently reconstrued in TT1, with the use of the conjunction "and" to link the two clause simplexes, indicating the extending relation of addition (+). In TT2, the translator chooses hypotaxis – his preferred choice – over parataxis. The preposition "for" in the non-Finite clause signals the enhancing relation of purpose (×).

Figure 4.4 shows the frequency of logico-semantic type in the analysis. Between the basic choice of expansion and projection, most choices are those of expansion, while only one choice of projection is seen in TT1 and TT2 respectively. From

Example 4.7, we find variations in terms of the choice of logico-semantic type in the ST and the two TTs (see Table 4.9). In the ST, the logico-semantic relation is that of extension (+), with the second clause adding more information to the two secret agents, extending the previous clause simplex by way of addition. In TT1, the logico-semantic relations of elaboration (+) and enhancement (×) are analyzed, which are characterized with the use of two non-Finite clauses. In TT2, besides

Table 4.9 Example 4.7

Tactic structure	ST	Tactic structure	TT1	Tactic structure	TT2
1	两 位 穿 灰色 大衫 的 – 宋恩子 与 吴祥子，正 低 声 地 谈话， PY: liǎng wèi chuān huī sè dà shān de – sòng ēn zi yǔ wú xiáng zi, zhèng dī shēng di tán huà, IG: two MEAS customer wear grey gown SUB Song Enzi and Wu Xiangzi, VPART low voice VPART talk BT: Two men in grey gowns – Song Enzi and Wu Xiangzi are now talking in a low voice.	α	Song Enzi and Wu Xiangzi, <<wearing grey gowns,>> are talking secretively.	–	Two men in grey gowns, Song Enz and Wu Xiangzi, are talking to each other in whispers.
+2	看样子他们是北 衙 门 的 办案的（侦缉）。 PY: kàn yàng zi tā men shì běi yá men de bàn àn de (zhēn jī) IG: seem they be north court SUB detective (spy) BT: It seems they are detectives (spies) from the north court.	=β	<<wearing grey gowns,>>	α	From their appearance one can deduce
		×β	Judging by their appearance	'β	they are agents from the Northern Yamen, the security authority in those days.
		α	they are police agents from the Northern Yamen.		

Source: Adapted from Lao (1999: 6–7, 2004: 12–15)

Table 4.10 Example 4.8

Tactic structure	ST	Tactic structure	TT1	Tactic structure	TT2
α	屋子 非常 高大, PY: wū zi fēi cháng gāo dà, IG: room very big BT: The room is very big.	–	The room should be large and high-ceilinged, with both oblong tables and square ones, and traditional teahouse benches and stools.	–	The building is extremely large and high, with rectangular tables, square tables, benches and stools for the customers.
+β	摆 着 长桌 与 方桌, 长凳 与 小凳, PY: bǎi zhe cháng zhuō yǔ fāng zhuō, cháng dèng yǔ xiǎo dèng, IG: put VPART rectangular table and square table bench and stool BT: Rectangular tables, square tables, benches and stools are put in the room.				
+γ	都 是 茶座儿。 PY: dōu shì chá zuò er IG: all be seat BT: Benches and stools are all seats.				

Source: Adapted from Lao (1999: 4–7, 2004: 12–13)

the omission of the extending relation (+) in the ST, the translator adds a mental process of "deduce," which projects a bound clause, leading to the addition of projection of thought (').

The preferred choice of logico-semantic type in the ST is extension (+), but these relations are seldom equivalently reconstrued in the TTs. In most cases, the relations are omitted by the translators when they combine several clause simplexes in the ST to one clause complex. For instance, in Example 4.8 (see Table 4.10), the prepositional phrases, such as "with both oblong tables and square ones, and traditional teahouse benches and stools" in TT1 and "with rectangular tables, square tables, benches and stools for the customers" in TT2 are used to translate the two clause simplexes with extending relations in the ST.

Enhancing relations (×) are frequently selected in TT1 and TT2. In most cases, they are translated from the enhancing relations in the ST. In Example 4.9 (see Table 4.11), the equivalent logico-semantic relations of enhancement (×) are found in the ST and both TTs. We also note that no conjunction such as "然后" (PY: rán hòu; IG: and then), which can mark out such temporal relation, is found

Table 4.11 Example 4.9

Tactic structure	ST	Tactic structure	TT1	Tactic structure	TT2
α	如某处的大蜘蛛怎么成了精， PY: rú mǒu chù de dà zhī zhū zěn me chéng le jīng, IG: such as some place SUB big spider how become ASP demon BT: such as how the big spider at some place becomes a demon.	α	such as how in a certain place a huge spider had turned into a demon	α	such as how a giant spider turned into a demon
×β	受到雷击。 PY: shòu dào léi jī IG: get thunder strike BT: got struck by thunder.	×β	and was then struck by lightning.	×β	until it was finally struck by lightning;

Source: Adapted from Lao (1999: 4–5, 2004: 12–13)

Table 4.12 Example 4.10

Tactic structure	ST	Tactic structure	TT1	Tactic structure	TT2
–	在这些条子旁边还贴着"茶钱先付"的新纸条。 PY: zài zhè xiē tiáo zi páng biān hái tiē zhe "chá qián xiān fù" de xīn zhǐ tiáo IG: CV these slip beside also paste VPART "tea money advance pay" SUB new paper slip BT: Beside these slips, there pastes new paper slip of "Pay tea money in advance"	1	Along with them there are some new notices:	–	Alongside these, new paper slips have been added, with "Please pay in advance" on them.
		=2	"Pay in advance."		

Source: Adapted from Lao (1999: 4–5, 2004: 12–13)

in the ST, while these relations are marked out explicitly by "and . . . then" in TT1 and "until" in TT2.

The frequency of elaborating relation (=) in the TTs is higher than that of the ST. Also, elaboration is the most frequently selected choice among all options in the system of LOGICO-SEMANTIC TYPE. In Example 4.10 (see Table 4.12), we find an elaborating relation (=) added in TT1, though no such relation is identified in the clause complex in the ST. In TT1, the second clause is a further exposition of the notice described in the first clause, resulting in the addition of the elaborating relation (=).

4.3   Tactic and logico-semantic type shift in stage direction

In translation, choices of taxis and logico-semantic type can be equivalent to those in the ST, as shown in Example 4.9, where the tactic structure and the logico-semantic relation are reconstrued equivalently in both TTs. However, equivalence within the logical metafunction cannot always be maintained. There have to be translation shifts to guarantee the equivalence elsewhere. In Sections 4.3.1 and 4.3.2, we will elaborate on the tactic and logico-semantic type shifts in detail.

4.3.1   Tactic shift in stage direction

Different types of tactic shift are summarized and quantified based on the categories of addition, omission, and substitution (see Table 4.13). The total frequencies of the tactic shift are similar, with TT2 outnumbering TT1 for one shift. The preferred type of tactic shift in TT2 is omission of parataxis, while the occurrences of the various subtypes of shifts in TT1 are even in general (except for substitution from hypotaxis to parataxis).

A larger number of additions of taxis (tactic additions) are found in TT1 than in TT2. These additions are related to the additions of clauses in the TTs, including both free clauses with Finites and non-Finite clauses. In Example 4.11 (see Table 4.14), the addition of a free clause in TT2, which is translated from "一清早" (PY: yì qīng zǎo; IG: one morning) that functions as a circumstance in the clause complex in the ST. By adding the clause simplex, a paratactic relation is added in TT2. An RST analysis reveals the same rhetorical structures in both TTs, which is multi-nucleus and addition (see Figure 4.5). In TT2, the paratactic relation is at the stratum of lexicogrammar, whereas in TT1, it is at the strata of semantics – a larger environment of translation in terms of stratification (Matthiessen 2001).

This is also illustrated with the stage direction about paper slips. The translator of TT1 has translated the content of the paper slips in the ST as free clauses. In the

Table 4.13 Different types of shift of taxis in the analysis of stage direction

Types of shift			*freq.in TT1*	*freq. in TT2*
tactic shift (shift of taxis)	addition	parataxis	5	2
		hypotaxis	5	3
	omission	parataxis	4	14
		hypotaxis	6	3
	substitution	from parataxis to hypotaxis	7	6
		from hypotaxis to parataxis	0	0
Total			27	28

Table 4.14 Example 4.11

Tactic structure	ST	Tactic structure	TT1	Tactic structure	TT2
–	一清早，还没有下窗板。 PY: yì qīng zǎo, hái méi yǒu xià chuāng bǎn IG: one morning, still NEG have remove window shutter BT: One morning, the window shutter have not been removed.	–	It is early in the morning.	1	It is early morning,
		–	The shutters have not yet been removed from the windows.	+2	the wooden shutters have not yet been taken down from the windows.

Source: Adapted from Lao (1999: 130–131, 2004: 112–113)

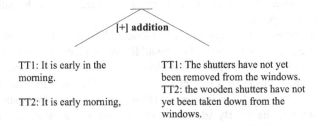

TT1: It is early in the morning.

TT2: It is early morning,

TT1: The shutters have not yet been removed from the windows.
TT2: the wooden shutters have not yet been taken down from the windows.

Figure 4.5 The rhetorical structures in TT1 and TT2 in Example 4.11

ST, these paper slips include "莫谈国事" (PY: mò tán guó shì; IG: NEG talk state affair) and "茶钱先付" (PY: chá qián xiān fù; IG: tea money advance pay), which are both embedded and function as Epithets in nominal groups. Example 4.10 illustrates (see Table 4.12) how a free clause, i.e. "Pay in advance," is added in TT1, leading to the addition of a paratactic relation of elaboration.

The reconstrual of the logical structures can also lead to tactic shifts. As previously shown in Example 4.5 (see Table 4.7), we find a hypotactic relation added in TT2 with the help of the last three clauses, i.e. "his shoes half off his feet," "and wearing an extremely long and dirty gown," and "some scraps of paper tucked into his hat near the temples" (Lao 1999: 9), all of which are non-Finite clauses that describe the appearance of Tang the Oracle. In the ST, however, such a depiction is found in the first three clauses. The process in the final clause in the ST – "进来" (PY: jìn lái; IG: enter) – is found in the first clause in both TTs.

In terms of omissions of taxis (tactic omissions), we find an especially large number of paratactic omissions in TT2, with a frequency of 14 (see Table 4.13). We also

Table 4.15 Example 4.12

Tactic structure	ST	Tactic structure	TT1	Tactic structure	TT2
×β	假若 有 什么 突出 惹 眼的 东西， PY: jiǎ ruò yǒu shén me tū chū rě yǎn de dōng xi, IG: if have some striking eye-catching thing BT: It there are any striking and eye-catching things,	–	The only thing that might catch the eye at all is the proliferation of "Don't discuss state affairs" notices . . .	×β	If there is anything outstanding [[which catches the eye]],
α	那 就 是 "莫 谈 国事" 的 纸条 更多， PY: nà jiù shì "mò tán guó shì" de zhǐ tiáo gèng duō, IG: that then be NEG talk state affair SUB paper slip more BT: then that is there are more paper slips of "Don't talk about state affairs"			α	it is the paper slips with "Do not discuss affairs of state" on them.

Source: Adapted from Lao (1999: 130–131, 2004: 110–111)

note that most of these omissions in TT2 are those of parataxis, while the omitted relations in TT1 are mainly the hypotactic ones. As illustrated in Example 4.12 (see Table 4.15), the hypotactic relation in the ST is omitted in TT1 when the translator combines the clause simplexes in the ST into one clause complex. However, in TT2, the translator has reconstrued the hypotactic relation equivalently.

Tactic omission is also related to the omission of clauses in the ST. As shown in Example 4.13 (see Table 4.16), the two clauses in the ST are linked hypotactically. In both TTs, the second clause in the ST, which contains a relational process, has been omitted. In TT1, the clause is left untranslated. In TT2, it is translated as "well-known for their physical prowess," a post-modifying element, specifically the Qualifier of the nominal group. In terms of rank in lexicogrammar, the shift in TT2 is from clause to group/phrase, i.e. shifting from a wide environment of translation to a narrow one in terms of rank (Matthiessen 2001).

Moreover, in TT1, the translator has omitted all of the three paratactic relations following "幕 启" (PY: mù qǐ) at the beginning of the three acts. For instance, in Example 4.14 (see Table 4.17), the first clause is translated and capitalized as "SCENE" in TT1, with the logical relations between the two clauses in the ST omitted. In TT2, we find that the paratactic relation is reconstrued equivalently.

Substitution of taxis (tactic substitution) includes both parataxis to hypotaxis and vice versa. According to the analysis, the substitutions in TT1 and TT2 are all

Table 4.16 Example 4.13

Tactic structure	ST	Tactic structure	TT1	Tactic structure	TT2
α	因为 被约的 打手 中 包括 着 善扑 营 的 哥 儿们 和 库兵， PY: yīn wéi bèi yuē de dǎ shǒu zhōng bāo kuò zhe shàn pū yíng de gē er men hé kù bīng, IG: because invited fighter in include VPART Wrestling Academy SUB brothers and storehouse guard BT: Because the invited fighters include brothers from the Wrestling Academy and guards of the Imperial Storehouse.	–	because vicious thugs from the Wrestling Academy and the Guards from the Imperial Storehouses had been hired.	–	for the toughs invited by both parties included characters well-known for their physical prowess such as the Imperial Wrestlers and Guards of the Imperial Storehouses.
+β	身手 都 十分 厉害。 PY: shēn shǒu dōu shí fēn lì hài IG: skill all very superb BT: their skills are all superb				

Source: Adapted from Lao (1999: 6–9, 2004: 14–15)

Table 4.17 Example 4.14

Tactic structure	ST	Tactic structure	TT1	Tactic structure	TT2
1	幕启： PY: mù qǐ IG: curtain rise BT: The curtain rises:	–	SCENE	1	The curtain rises:
+2	这 种 大 茶 馆 现在 已经 不 见 了。 PY: zhè zhǒng dà chá guǎn xiàn zài yǐ jīng bú jiàn le IG: this kind big teahouse now already NEG seen ASP BT: This kind of big teahouse is already not seen now.	–	Large teahouses like this are no longer to be seen	+2	One doesn't find large teahouses like this any more.

Source: Adapted from Lao (1999: 2–3, 2004: 10–11)

Table 4.18 Example 4.15

Tactic structure	ST	Tactic structure	TT1	Tactic structure	TT2
1	马五爷 在 不惹人注意的 角落, PY: mǎ wǔ yé zài bù rě rén zhù yì de jiǎo luò, IG: Master Ma CV inconspicuous corner BT: Master Ma is in an inconspicuous corner.	α	Fifth Elder Ma sits by himself in an inconspicuous corner	α	Master Ma, alone in a corner, sits inconspicuously
+2	独自 坐 着 PY: dú zì zuò zhe IG: alone sit VPART BT: Master Ma sits alone.	=β	drinking tea.	=β	drinking tea.
+3	喝 茶。 PY: hē chá IG: drink tea BT: Master Ma drinks tea.				

Source: Adapted from Lao (1999: 8–9, 2004: 14–15)

from parataxis to hypotaxis, which are associated with the use of non-Finite clauses. In Example 4.15 (see Table 4.18), the paratactic structure in the ST is changed to hypotaxis in both TTs, characterized with the use of non-Finite clauses – "drinking tea." Such dependent clauses add a further description to Master Ma, a character that is already fully specified in the previous dominant clause.

4.3.2 *Logico-semantic type shift in stage direction*

Table 4.19 tabulates and quantifies the types of logico-semantic type shift in both TTs. The total occurrences of logico-semantic type shift between the two TTs are similar, with five more shifts found in TT1. Similar to the way we discussed tactic shift in Section 4.3.1, we also describe the shifts of logico-semantic type in terms of addition, omission, and substitution. For both TTs, omissions of logico-semantic type have the largest occurrences among the three types of shift, while substitutions rank as second most frequent. Between expansion and projection, two choices in the system of LOGICO-SEMANTIC TYPE, most shifts of logico-semantic type are related to expansion. Further, we notice that projection is only involved in the addition of logico-semantic type rather than omission and substitution, with only one occurrence found in each TT.

Additions of logico-semantic type are generally related to the additions of clauses in the TTs. As previously shown in Example 4.7 (see Table 4.9), the additional clause in TT1, marked by the addition of "deduce" – a mental process – has resulted in the addition of projection of idea, which is a logico-semantic type not found in the ST.

Table 4.19 Different types of logico-semantic type shift in the analysis of stage direction

Types of shift		*freq. in TT1*	*freq. in TT2*
addition	elaboration (=)	4	0
	extension (+)	1	2
	enhancement (×)	2	2
	idea (')	1	1
	locution (")	0	0
omission	elaboration (=)	2	3
	extension (+)	21	21
	enhancement (×)	7	4
	locution (")	0	0
	idea (')	0	0
substitution	from extension (+) to elaboration (=)	6	6
	from extension (+) to enhancement (×)	3	3
	from enhancement (×) to elaboration (=)	2	0
	from enhancement (×) to extension (+)	0	1
	from elaboration (=) to extension (+)	0	1
Total		49	44

Also, translators may adopt a different way of clause complexing in contrast to the choices made in the ST. In Example 4.16 (see Table 4.20), the translator of TT2 has translated the two clause complexes in the ST as one clause complex, resulting in the addition of an extending relation (+). In TT1, the logico-semantic types in the ST are mostly maintained, except for an omission of the final enhancing relation (×) in the ST.

Omissions of logico-semantic type are associated with the omission of clauses in the TTs (see Example 4.17) and the translators' different choices of clause complexing (see Example 4.18). In Example 4.17 (see Table 4.21), omissions of "也 就够了" (PY: yě jiù gòu le; IG: also VADV enough ASP) are found in both TTs, with the hypotactic structure and enhancing relation (×) being meanwhile omitted.

In Example 4.18 (see Table 4.22), three clause complexes are used in TT2 to translate one clause complex in the ST. Thus, all logico-semantic relations in the ST are omitted, including an elaborating one (=) and an enhancing one (×).

Five combinations of logico-semantic type of substitution are found in the analysis, with the most frequent subtype of substitution being from extension (+) to elaboration (=) and all involving the use of non-Finite dependent clauses in the TTs. As shown in Example 4.19 (see Table 4.23), the logico-semantic type in the ST is extension (+), where a conjunction in Chinese such as "并且" (PY: bìng qiě; IG: and) or "而且" (PY: ér qiě; IG: and) can be added, though not necessary. In both TTs, however, we find non-Finite dependent clauses that add certain specific meanings to the previous clause.

Table 4.20 Example 4.16

Tactic structure	ST	Tactic structure	TT1	Tactic structure	TT2
1	在 这里，可以 听 到 最 荒唐 的 新闻， PY: zài zhè lǐ, kě yǐ tīng dào zuì huāng táng de xīn wén, IG: CV here can hear PV most ridiculous news BT: Here, one can hear the most ridiculous news.	1	In the teahouse, one could hear the most absurd stories,	1 α	At its tables one could hear the most preposterous stories,
=2 α	如 某 处 的 大 蜘蛛 怎么 成 了 精， PY: rú mǒu chù de dà zhī zhū zěn me chéng le jīng, IG: such as some place SUB big spider how become ASP demon BT: Such as a big spider at some place has become a demon.	=2 α	such as how in a certain place a huge spider had turned into a demon	1 =β α	such as how a giant spider turned into a demon
=2 ×β	受 到 雷 击。 PY: shòu dào léi jī IG: receive PV thunder BT The big spider was struck by thunder.	=2 ×β	and was then struck by lightning.	1 =β ×β	until it was finally struck by lightning;
1	奇怪 的 意见 也 在 这里 可以 听 到， PY qí guài de yì jiàn yě zài zhè lǐ kě yǐ tīng dào, IG strange view also CV here can hear PV BT Strange views can also be heard here.	1	One could also come in contact with the strangest views;	+2 α	or [one could hear] the most extraordinary views,
=2 ×β	像 把 海边 上 都 修 上 大 墙， PY: xiàng bǎ hǎi biān shàng dōu xiū shàng dà qiáng, IG: be like PASS seaside all build PV big wall BT: Such as one can build high walls on the seaside.	=2	for example, that foreign troops could be prevented from landing by building a Great Wall along the sea coast.	+2 =β	such as how far it was possible to prevent all foreign armies from landing by the simple expedient of building a long high wall along the seacoast.
=2 α	就 足以 挡住 洋 兵 上岸。 PY: jiù zú yǐ dǎng zhù yáng bīng shàng àn IG: VADV enough prevent foreign troop land BT: That is enough to prevent foreign troops from landing				

Source: Adapted from Lao (1999: 4–5, 2004: 12–13)

Table 4.21 Example 4.17

Tactic structure	ST	Tactic structure	TT1	Tactic structure	TT2
1	一进门 是 柜台 与 炉灶 – PY: yí jìn mén shì guì tái yǔ lú zào IG: entrance be counter and stove BT: At the entrance there is the counter and the stove.	1	Just inside the main entrance is the counter and a cookstove,	1	Immediately inside the entrance we see the counter and the brick stove,
×2×β	为 省 点 事, PY: wèi shěng diǎn shì, IG: to save some matter BT: To make things simple,	+2×β	to make things simpler,	×2α	though for the stage we can do away with the stove
×2α	我们的 舞台 上 可以 不 要 炉灶; PY: wǒ mén de wǔ tái shàng kě yǐ bú yào lú zào; IG: our stage on can NEG want stove BT: On our stage, we can have no stove.	+2α	the stove can be dispensed with	×2×β	if it's too much trouble
+3×β	后面 有些 锅 勺 的 响声 PY: hòu miàn yǒu xiē guō sháo de xiǎng shēng IG: back have some pot pan SUB sound BT: At the back there are some sounds of pots and pans.	+2×γ	if the clatter of pots and pans is heard off stage.	+3	and make do with the clatter of pots and pans offstage.
+3α	也 就 够 了。 PY: yě jiù gòu le IG: also VADV enough ASP BT: That is then enough.				

Source: Adapted from Lao (1999: 4–5, 2004: 12–13)

Table 4.22 Example 4.18

Tactic structure	ST	Tactic structure	TT1	Tactic structure	TT2
1	今天 又 有 一 起 打群架 的, PY: jīn tiān yòu yǒu yì qǐ dǎ qún jià de, IG: today again have one MEAS fighting BT: Today in the teahouse, there is again one fighting.	1	Today, another quarrel has broken out between two gangs;	–	Another gang fight has been brewing today.

Tactic structure	ST	Tactic structure	TT1	Tactic structure	TT2
=2	据说 是 为了 争 一 只 家 鸽， PY: jù shuō shì wèi le zhēng yì zhī jiā gē, IG: allegedly be for take one MEAS pigeon BT: It is said to be over a pigeon.	=2	the dispute is said to be over a pigeon.	–	The reason, according to some sources, was a dispute over the ownership of a pigeon.
×3	惹起 非 用 武力 解决 不 可 的 纠纷。 PY: rě qǐ fēi yòng wǔ lì jiě jué bù kě de jiū fēn IG: cause must use force solve NEG can SUB dispute BT: That caused dispute that has to be solved by force.	–	It seemed that it could not be settled without resort to violence, . . .	–	It seemed quite likely that the whole affair might end in violence.

Source: Adapted from Lao (1999: 6–7, 2004: 14–15)

Table 4.23 Example 4.19

Tactic structure	ST	Tactic structure	TT1	Tactic structure	TT2
1	藤椅 已 不 见， PY: téng yǐ bú jiàn, IG: wicker chair already NEG seen BT: The wicker chairs are already not seen,	α	The wicker chairs are gone,	α	The wicker chairs have disappeared,
+2	代 以 小凳 与 条凳。 PY: dài yǐ xiǎo dèng yǔ tiáo dèng IG: replace by stool and bench BT: replaced by stools and benches.	=β	having been replaced with stools and benches.	=β	replaced by stools and benches.

Source: Adapted from Lao (1999: 130–131, 2004: 110–111)

The translators can purposely choose a different logico-semantic type to substitute the one in the ST. According to Example 4.20 (see Table 4.24), the extending relation (+) is changed to an enhancing one (×) in TT2, which indicates the purpose of removing the stove. In TT1, the logico-semantic type in the ST is reconstrued equivalently, both being additive extensions (+) that link the two clause simplexes.

Table 4.24 Example 4.20

Tactic structure	ST	Tactic structure	TT1	Tactic structure	TT2
1	厨房 挪 到 后面 去， PY: chú fáng nuó dào hòu miàn qù, IG: kitchen move PV back PV BT: The kitchen is moved to the back,	1	The kitchen has been moved out back,	α	The stove has been removed to the back,
+2	专 包 公寓住客 的伙食。 PY: zhuān bāo gōng yù zhù kè de huǒ shí IG: especially serve lodger SUB meal BT: especially serves lodger's meals	+2	and only serves meals for the lodgers.	×β	for preparing meals for the lodgers.

Source: Adapted from Lao (1999: 58–59, 2004: 54–55)

4.4 Summary

In this chapter, we analyzed and compared the logical choices made in the stage direction of *Teahouse*, involving the analysis in systems of TAXIS and LOGICO-SEMANTIC TYPE. We observed some quantitative similarities and differences and examined two translation shifts within the logical metafunction, i.e. tactic shift and logico-semantic type shift (Matthiessen 2014b). Delicate categories of these shifts, such as tactic addition, omission, and substitution, were discussed, and the preferred patterns of these shifts were pointed out.

Stage direction, as one necessary component in *Teahouse*, has seldom been considered in previous studies (e.g. Ren 2008; Guo & Ding 2009; Shen 2010; Peng 2013). By pointing out the logical choices made by the playwright and the two translators, the analysis in this chapter not only fills this research gap but also helps us understand the choices made in the translation of stage direction – texts in which reporting and enabling fields of activity are recreated (see Section 5.3). In addition, different choices among the two translators were observed. The translator of TT2, who tends to adopt a "free" strategy of translation in dramatic dialogue and dramatic monologue, has not made many changes to the stage direction from the logical perspective. In terms of the frequency of tactic shift and logico-semantic type shift, we found a similar occurrence of tactic shift in both TTs and a lesser frequency of logico-semantic type shift in TT2 (see Table 4.13 and Table 4.19).

Some typological similarities and differences between English and Chinese can be seen based on the lexicogrammatical analysis of taxis and logico-semantic type.

First, the choices in the systems of TAXIS and LOGICO-SEMANTIC TYPE are mostly the same in English and Chinese (cf. Figure 4.1). The choice of hypotactic elaboration ($\alpha=\beta$), however, has not been found in our analysis of the Chinese ST, nor has it been described in Li's (2007) descriptive work on Mandarin Chinese. Besides, in the English TTs, we find a large number of such hypotactic elaborations realized by non-Finite dependent clauses – an option not available in Chinese.

Second, in the Chinese ST, we find various markers of the logico-semantic relations in our data. For elaborating relations, there are markers like "如" (PY: rú; IG: be like) and "像" (PY: xiàng; IG: be like). For extending relations, such markers include "也" (PY: yě; IG: and), "而" (PY: ér; IG: and), "并" (PY: bìng; IG: and), "而且" (PY: ér qiě; IG: and), "不但 . . . 而且" (PY: bú dàn . . . ér qiě; IG: not only . . . but also), and "但是" (PY: dàn shì; IG: but). Also, markers of enhancing relation include "假若" (PY: jiǎ ruò; IG: if), "以期" (PY: yǐ qī; IG: in order to), "因为" (PY: yīn wéi; IG: because), "可是" (PY: kě shì; IG: but), and "却" (PY: què; IG: but). In the English TTs, these markers are translated explicitly.

Third, omissions of such markers, most of which are conjunctions, are found both in the ST and the TTs. In the ST, such omissions are more commonly seen, thereby increasing the difficulty in analyzing the ST.

Different from dramatic dialogue and dramatic monologue, stage direction is unique in that it is not translated to be spoken or read aloud. During the translation process, the primary focus of the translators is on the experiential meaning rather than the logical, interpersonal, and textual meanings. However, our analysis in this chapter highlights the logical choices that translators have to make. Based on the analysis, there are some implications for translation practice.

First, a translator may choose to reconstrue the logical meaning equivalently or not. If an equivalent logical choice is required, he will first need to interpret the logical choices in the Chinese ST and then find the equivalent ones in the English TT.

Second, some logical choices, such as the use of the logical connectors and markers of the logico-semantic relations, are associated with the lexicogrammatical resources of COHESION, involving the system of CONJUNCTION (Halliday & Hasan 1976). When translating stage direction from Chinese to English, a translator can choose to translate the conjunctions explicitly or implicitly. He or she can also choose to translate the implicit conjunctions in the ST explicitly.

Third, coupled with analysis of textual meaning, we can find other possibilities of translation shifts from textual metafunction to logical or vice versa (see Wang 2017). For instance, translation shifts from textual to logical will occur when implicit textual transitions in the ST are made explicit in the TT. Conversely, we will find translation shifts from logical to textual when the tactically related clauses in the ST are translated as structurally unrelated ones, leaving the tactic structures for readers to infer (see Matthiessen 2014b; Wang & Ma 2018). However, it must be noted that these shifts, different from errors, are inevitable in that the translators may shift here to gain equivalence elsewhere (Halliday 2010). Equivalence is thus likely to be maintained in a larger environment of translation (Matthiessen 2001), such as semantics or context in terms of stratification, clause rank in terms of rankscale in lexicogrammar, system in terms of axis, and less delicate systemic choice in terms of delicacy (see Figure 1.3).

5   Analyzing field, tenor, and mode

Perspectives from context

In this chapter, we move from lexicogrammar to context and investigate the data of dramatic dialogue, dramatic monologue, and stage direction from the perspectives of the three contextual parameters, i.e. field, tenor, and mode. First, we identify similarities and differences between the ST and the two TTs in these three aspects and relate this to our lexicogrammatical analysis in Chapters 2, 3, and 4. The contextual analysis provides evidence for the lexicogrammatical choices discussed in Chapters 2, 3, and 4, as the translators' choices are to some extent influenced by context.

5.1   The three contextual parameters in Systemic Functional Linguistics

Text, as language functioning in context, is located in the stratum of semantics as the highest unit on the rank scale. Context, as a higher-order semiotic system located above the linguistic system, is theorized as a stratum above semantics. The relationship between text and context is dynamic and reversible in that texts reveal context, and context is realized in texts (Butt et al. 1994). On the one hand, knowledge about context helps us predict the lexicogrammar of the text. On the other hand, lexicogrammatical analysis helps us understand context, as the total meaning encoded in lexicogrammar will become the sign of context (Halliday 1978, 1991a; Halliday & Hasan 1985).

Notions of context date back to the works by Malinowski (e.g. 1923) and Firth (e.g. 1957) (Butt & Wegener 2007; Hasan 2009). These works have been further developed in linguistics by Halliday and others in different linguistic traditions. In SFL, context is not only theorized in terms of the dimension of stratification but is also modeled along the cline of instantiation. The relationship between context of culture and context of situation is similar to relationship between system (meaning potential) and text (instance). Context of culture, which "defines the potential, or range of possibilities available in language as a system" is located at the system pole of the cline of instantiation (Halliday 1978: 55). Context of situation, which is "specified with respect to field, tenor and mode," and "plays a significant role in determining the actual choices among these possibilities," is located at the instance pole of the cline (ibid.).

The three contextual parameters or variables include field, tenor, and mode, which are "highly general concepts for describing how the context of situation determines the kinds of meaning that are expressed" (Halliday & Hasan 1985: 12). The semiotic systems of FIELD, TENOR, and MODE have been explained as follows.

> The FIELD OF DISCOURSE refers to what is happening, to the nature of the social action that is taking place: what is it that the participants are engaged in, in which the language figures as some essential component?
>
> The TENOR OF DISCOURSE refers to who is taking part, to the nature of the participants, their statuses and roles: what kinds of role relationship obtain among the participants, including permanent and temporary relationships of one kind or another, both the types of speech role that they are taking on in the dialogue and the whole cluster of socially significant relationships in which they are involved.
>
> The MODE OF DISCOURSE refers to what part the language is playing, what it is that the participants are expecting the language to do for them in that situation: the symbolic organization of the text, the status that it has, and its function in the context, including the channel (is it spoken or written or some combination of the two?) and also the rhetorical mode, what is being achieved by the text in terms of such categories as persuasive, expository, didactic, and the like.
>
> (ibid.)

The contextual analysis in this chapter takes all three parameters into consideration. In terms of field, we examine the ST and the TTs based on Matthiessen's (e.g. 2015a, 2015b, 2015c) field of activity, which characterizes texts contextually from the perspective of the eight **socio-semiotic processes**, including "expounding," "reporting," "recreating," "sharing," "doing," "enabling," "recommending," and "exploring" (see Figure 5.1). The eight primary fields of activities can be grouped into three major categories: process of meaning (semiotic processes), process of behaving (social processes), and transition between the two (semiotic processes potentially leading to social processes). These social-semiotic processes can all be extended with delicacy into various subtypes. The definitions of the fields of activity are as follows (see Matthiessen 2015c: 55–56):

> **semiotic processes** (i.e. "meaning" processes – semiotic processes constitutive of context, constituted as semiotic processes and manifested through social processes):
>
> • **expounding** knowledge about general classes of phenomena (rather than particular instances of phenomena), theorizing our experience of the world in terms of a commonsense (folk) or uncommonsense (scientific) model by explaining why general classes of events take place or by categorizing general classes of entities (in terms of taxonomies, hyponymic and/or meronymic, and/or characterization);
> • **reporting** on particular instances of phenomena (rather than general classes of phenomena) creating "episodic" knowledge (rather than

theoretical knowledge), the type of reporting being dependent on the nature of the phenomena: chronicling (the flow of) particular events, inventorying particular entities, or surveying particular places;

- **recreating** various aspects of life – involving any of the eight different types of context according to field of activity, typically imagined (fictional) rather than experienced (factual: experienced personally or vicariously), as verbal art with a "theme" (in the sense of Hasan 1985), through narration and/or dramatization;
- **sharing** personal experiences and values (opinions, attitudes, feelings) as part of establishing, maintaining, and calibrating, (in short, negotiating) interpersonal relationships – in terms of the tenor of the relationship among interactants, ranging from (and potentially transforming) stranger-hood to intimacy but sustained over longer periods of time, involving fairly intimate relationships in different institutions such as kinship and friendship; in terms of mode, traditionally and prototypically in private face-to-face interaction but increasingly enabled by new technologies opening up new channels of sharing (epistolary, telegraphic, telephonic – and now with an explosion of mobile and Internet based possibilities, with a tendency to blur the distinction between private and public spheres);
- **exploring** public values (opinions, stances) and positions (ideas, hypotheses) by reviewing commodities (assigning them values on a scale from very positive to very negative) or by arguing about positions, debating or discussing them – in terms of tenor, typically between one person (a professional or a member of the general public) and some segment of the general public, so between strangers; in terms of mode, typically using media channels, either "old" media channels (print, radio, TV) or "new" media channels (mobile and/or Internet-based);

semiotic processes potentially leading to social processes (i.e. "meaning" leading to "doing"):

- **recommending** some course of action (typically some kind of social process – exhortation in the strong form), either for the sake of the addressees by advising them to undertake it for their own good or for the sake of the speaker by promoting some type of goods-&-services;
- **enabling** some course of action (typically some kind of social process), either literally enabling (empowering) them by instructing them in some type of procedure or constraining them by regulating their behavior;

social processes (i.e. "doing" processes – social processes constitutive of context, semiotic processes facilitating [i.e. "meaning" facilitating "doing"]):

- **doing** – performing some form of social behavior, on one's own or as part of a team, with semiotic processes ("meaning") coming in to facilitate this social behavior through direction or collaboration.

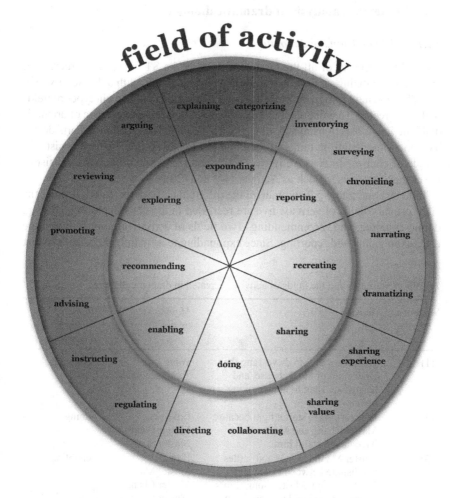

Figure 5.1 The eight primary fields of activity and their subtypes

Source: Matthiessen, Wang & Ma (2019: 99)

Our description of tenor is carried out in two aspects, including (i) tenor relations between the playwright/translators and the readers and (ii) tenor relations between the various characters in the play. We will analyze *Teahouse* and its two translations in terms of institutional roles, power and status roles, and distance between the ST and two TTs. In terms of mode, our analysis is conducted from the perspectives of rhetorical mode, medium, channel, orientation, and turn-ranking. Taken together, the analysis of field, tenor, and mode will define the context of situation of the ST and the TTs and will contribute to our understanding of the lexicogrammatical properties of the texts. The next three sections in this chapter will each focus on the contextual analysis of one of the three text types in *Teahouse*.

5.2 Contextual analysis of dramatic dialogue

5.2.1 Field of dramatic dialogue

The field of activity of all the three text types in the ST is primarily recreating through dramatizing, and the activities here are imagined, with a theme of verbal art. When the field falls in the category of recreating, one of the eight types of fields will be recreated. To point out these recreated fields, we divide the data of dramatic dialogue into 22 sections in accordance with the plot. These different parts do not have the same length in terms of the number of clauses. Some parts consist of a couple of clauses, such as Activity (1), (2), and (3), while other parts consist of fewer than ten clauses, such as Activity (14) and (20).

Table 5.1 and Table 5.2 summarize the different activity recreated. Among the eight primary fields of activity, five are recreated in the data: exploring, sharing, doing, enabling, and recommending. Two fields of activity are not found in the data: expounding and reporting. Since expounding texts mainly theorize, explain,

Table 5.1 Activities and the fields of activity recreated in dramatic dialogue

Sequence	Activity	Major characters involved	Field of activity recreated
(1)	Wang Lifa tries to drive Tang the Oracle out of the teahouse, and he advises Tang to quit smoking opium.	Wang Lifa, Tang the Oracle	enabling
(2)	Erdez wants to start a fight because Master Chang and Master Song have talked about him.	Erdez, Master Chang, Master Song	doing
(3)	Master Ma intervenes and settles the dispute between Erdez and Master Chang. Master Song wants to pay for the bowl that has been broken during the fight.	Erdez, Master Ma, Master Chang, Master Song	enabling
(4)	Master Chang laments that the silver in the empire is flowing out to foreign countries after trying the snuff offered by Pock-Mark Liu.	Master Chang, Pock-Mark Liu	sharing
(5)	Pock-Mark Liu threatens Kang Liu to sell Kang's daughter, Kang Shunz.	Pock-Mark Liu, Kang Liu	enabling
(6)	Pock-Mark Liu discusses his filthy business with Master Chang and Master Song. Master Chang despises the human trafficking business.	Pock-Mark Liu, Master Chang, Master Song	sharing
(7)	Pock-Mark Liu sells a tiny watch to Master Song.	Pock-Mark Liu, Master Song	doing
(8)	Tubby Huang comes in the teahouse to settle a dispute and is led to the backyard.	Tubby Huang, Wang Lifa	enabling

Sequence	Activity	Major characters involved	Field of activity recreated
(9)	An old-aged vendor comes in, and discusses the fight in the backyard with Li San and Master Song, and comments on affairs of state.	Li San, Master Song, old-aged vendor	exploring
(10)	The landowner of the teahouse, Master Qin, comes in and demands an increase in the rent. Wang Lifa tries to ingratiate himself with Master Qin.	Master Qin, Wang Lifa	sharing
(11)	A peasant woman tries to sell her starving little daughter. Wang Lifa wants to drive them out by following Master's Qin's suggestion. Master Chang then buys the mother and daughter noodles to fill their empty stomachs.	Master Qin, Wang Lifa, Master Chang	doing
(12)	Master Qin expresses his wish of starting a factory and saving the empire by engaging in industry.	Master Qin, Wang Lifa	sharing
(13)	Master Qin and Eunuch Pang greet each other.	Master Qin, Eunuch Pang	sharing
(14)	Eunuch Pang looks for Pock-Mark Liu, and Liu gives Eunuch Pang his regards.	Pock-Mark Liu, Eunuch Pang	sharing
(15)	Some customers in the teahouse discuss state affairs and express their views on the reform that just ended in failure.	other customers	sharing
(16)	Pock-Mark Liu tries to sell Kang Liu's daughter to Eunuch Pang and discusses the price with him.	Pock-Mark Liu, Eunuch Pang	recommending
(17)	Tang the Oracle returns to the teahouse, because soldiers are arresting reformers in the street. Tang greets Eunuch Pang.	Tang the Oracle, Eunuch Pang	sharing
(18)	Master Chang and Master Song are arrested by Song Enz and Wu Xiangz because of discussing state affairs.	Song Enz, Wu Xiangz, Master Chang, Master Song	doing
(19)	Tubby Huang refuses to help Master Chang and Master Song.	Tubby Huang	sharing
(20)	Tubby Huang greets Eunuch Pang and congratulates him on his marriage.	Tubby Huang, Eunuch Pang	sharing
(21)	The peasant woman decides not to sell her little daughter, so they leave the teahouse.	peasant woman	doing
(22)	Kang Liu sells his daughter, Shunz, to Eunuch Pang.	Kang Liu	doing

Table 5.2 Fields of activity being recreated in dramatic dialogue

Field of activity recreated	Sequence of the activity
sharing	(4) (6) (10) (13) (14) (15) (17) (19) (20)
doing	(2) (7) (11) (18) (21) (22)
enabling	(1) (3) (5) (8)
exploring	(9) (12)
recommending	(16)

or categorize knowledge, and reporting texts mainly report on particular instances of phenomena by chronicling, inventorying, or surveying, Lao She does not recreate them in the dramatization of events in Act One of *Teahouse*, which mostly consists of conversations between customers in the teahouse.

The exploring and sharing fields of activity are two semiotic processes that are both processes of meaning. One occurrence of exploring activity is found, which involves Li San and the Old Man's stance on aged people. In terms of tenor, the relationship between the characters involved in the exploring field of activity is strangers that meet for the first time.

In addition, the characters can share their values or experiences in the sharing field of activity. Nine instances are found, which have the largest frequency among the five fields of activity here recreated in the data. Examples include Master Chang sharing his attitude toward human trafficking with his friend Master Song and Pock-Mark Liu – the human trafficker – and Master Qin sharing his values of saving the empire through engaging in industry with Wang Lifa. In both cases, the people involved are acquaintances rather than complete strangers.

There are social processes of doing that entail social behaviors, and semiotic processes are used to facilitate the social processes. Six instances of doing field of activity are found, which include social behaviors of fighting, transaction (buying and selling), and arrest. Most of the doing activities are transactions, especially those of human trafficking in the teahouse. Some transactions are successful, such as Pock-Mark Liu selling the watch to Master Song and Kang Liu selling his daughter to Eunuch Pang. One transaction fails, as the peasant woman regrets selling her daughter and leaves the teahouse.

There are also semiotic processes that potentially lead to social processes, i.e. recommending and enabling, which both serve as transactions between social and semiotic processes. One recommending field of activity is found – Pock-Mark Liu trying to sell Kang Liu's daughter to Eunuch Pang, i.e. to provide goods and services by way of promoting. Four enabling fields of activity are found. One example is Wang Lifa's way of regulating Tang the Oracle's behavior; another example is Pock-Mark Liu's instruction to Kang Liu for selling his daughter.

In the two TTs, we find all recreated fields equivalently translated. No field has been added or omitted. The analysis of field sketches the major events in the plot and provides a basis for the analysis of tenor.

5.2.2 Tenor of dramatic dialogue

As previously discussed, the descriptions of tenor in the dramatic dialogue and dramatic monologue are twofold, as there are characters involved in these two types of text.

5.2.2.1 Tenor between the playwright/translators and the readers

First, in terms of institutional role, Lao She (the writer of the ST) is a famous Chinese playwright and novelist. He used to teach in various schools and universities both in China and abroad. As a patriot, he returned to China in 1950 after the People's Republic of China was established and was soon appointed important positions in major literary organizations (Tam 2004: xxxiii). In his works written in this period, including *Teahouse*, he continued to praise the socialist achievements and the new life brought to the common people by the country (Hu 1980; Zhang 2000).

The translator of TT1, John Howard-Gibbon, used to be a journalist and a college teacher of English language and literature in China. The motivations for him to translate *Teahouse* included his interest in Chinese language, his love for Chinese literature, and his desire to improve his proficiency in Chinese (Howard-Gibbon 2004; Mackenzie 2011).

Ying Ruocheng, the translator of TT2, was a professional actor of Beijing People's Art Theatre, where *Teahouse* was first performed. It is also noted that Ying has played the character of Pock-Mark Liu on stage. By the time he translated *Teahouse*, John Howard-Gibbon's translation had already been published. Ying believed that John Howard-Gibbon's translation was error-ridden, with many cultural connotations wrongly translated (see Howard-Gibbon 2004). In addition, he held that the already-made translation was not suitable for performance (Ying 1999; cf. Ying & Conceison 2009). Thus, he wanted to provide a concise and colloquial translation.

Second, for power and status roles, the roles between Lao She and the audience and Howard-Gibbon and the audience as well as Ying Ruocheng and the audience are unequal. They all adopt the role of a recounter and are responsible for characterization, i.e. depiction of the various characters in the play. The complementary role is assigned to the audience or readers.

Third, in terms of distance, the playwright and the translators are authorities, both as persons holding the authority and as specialists of the career, whereas the readers and the audience are unseen and unknown.

Before the play was shown on stage, Lao She tried to reduce the distance between him and his audience, so he consulted the various actors and directors from Beijing People's Art Theatre and made several revisions based on their suggestions (see Liu 2007). Ying Ruocheng, the translator of TT2, also attempted to bridge this distance. He emphasized performability and thus used colloquial and concise language to help audiences to understand the play. However, no similar attempt was made by John Howard-Gibbon, as his focus was mainly on the accuracy of the translation. In his own words, his limited fluency in the language forced him to "dwell over the text" and had made him very "text sensitive" (Howard-Gibbon 2004).

Since drama is a special text type that involves the presence of an audience that plays an eavesdropping role (cf. Halliday 1994b), we have to pay attention to the tenor relations between the translators and the audience. As the relations between John Howard-Gibbon, Ying Ruocheng, and the audience are unequal, the translators have both adopted the role of a recounter and are thus free to make changes in their choices. Their choices of mood have reflected such tenor relations. As reflected in our lexicogrammatical analysis in Chapter 2, we note that mood shifts are extensively found in both TTs – sometimes even the speech functions in the ST are changed (see Table 2.6, Examples 2.52, 2.53, 2.54). Quantitatively, similar occurrences of mood shifts are found in the TTs, while the frequency in TT1 is slightly higher. Some patterns for such changes in the translations are found, for example, mood shifts from declarative to imperative (see Example 2.6). Theoretically, all combinations of mood shifts may occur, but some substitutions are not found in our data, while some substitutions are found with a higher frequency (see Table 2.6), such as mood shifts from imperative to declarative (see Examples 2.51, 2.52, 2.53) and mood shifts from interrogative to declarative (see Example 2.54).

5.2.2.2 *Tenor between characters in the play*

In the analysis of the tenor of the recreated context, we examine the relationship between the main characters in Act One of *Teahouse*. The characters in *Teahouse* are representative, reflecting various people from different social hierarchies of the time (Ying 1999; Liu 2007). In Table 5.3, we provide a brief profile of these characters and list some of their general information, such as institutional role, age, and personality. We have also translated Lao She's comments on the characters into English (see e.g. Liu 2007: 308–309), since this reflects the playwright's perception of the major characters.

In the following paragraphs, we discuss the social statuses of the major characters based on the analysis of mood choices in Section 2.2 in the first act of the play. This will enable an understanding of the relationship between the characters.

Pock-Mark Liu, a human trafficker who sells children and women to the rich, is a malicious character in the play. He also has different strategies when talking to people with different statuses. When speaking to Kang Liu and Kang Shunz, who have lower statuses, he is remorseless. According to the analysis of mood in the ST, Pock-Mark Liu has contributed the largest number of interrogatives among all characters. Furthermore, he uses a lot of imperatives, and most of these interrogatives and imperatives are addressed to Kang Liu, realizing the speech functions of "question" and "command." Some imperatives are also addressed to Master Song to invite him to purchase a tiny watch. However, while speaking to Eunuch Pang, who is the buyer of Kang Liu's daughter, only declaratives are found among all of Pock-Mark Liu's free clauses. In the TTs, the interrogatives in the ST tend to be translated as declaratives to add more certainty to Pock-Mark Liu's assertions

Table 5.3 Some general information about the characters in Act One of *Teahouse*

Name	Age	Gender	Institutional role	Personality and extra information	Lao She's comment on the character	English translation of Lao She's comment
Wang Lifa	a little over 20	male	manager of Yutai Teahouse	his father died early, a shrewd man, somewhat selfish, but not really bad at heart	真真假假 千变万化 只求保暖 太平天下	As a hypocritical and capricious man, all he wants is a sheltered life and some peaceful time.
Pock-Mark Liu	in his thirties	male	professional pimp	vile and venomous	贩卖人口 一世缺德 别人落泪 他吃他喝	As a human trafficker, he does despicable business to prosper. While others shed tears, he is having a sumptuous dinner.
Master Chang	around 30	male	Manchurian, regular customer at Yutai Teahouse, good friend of Master Song	upright and robust	说打就打 有些骨气 直言无隐 哪怕入大狱	As a man of integrity, he fights when necessary. He also speaks bluntly and is sent to prison for this.
Qin Zhongyi	in his twenties	male	owner of the teahouse	son of a rich family, capitalist with reformist leanings	富国裕民 振兴实业 自己发财 目空一切	To make the empire and its people rich, to develop an industry is his wish. Being a wealthy man, he is as proud as he can be.
Kang Liu	around 40 years old	male	a starving peasant, father of Kang Shunz	bankrupted, lives in the outskirts of Beijing	国乱民贫 农村破产 卖女卖儿 苟延残喘	The empire is in a mess, and its people are penniless. Parents prolong their death throes by selling their boys and girls.
Master Song	in his thirties	male	Manchurian, regular customer at Yutai Teahouse, good friend of Master Chang	timid and talkative	—	—

(Continued)

Table 5.3 (Continued)

Name	Age	Gender	Institutional role	Personality and extra information	Lao She's comment on the character	English translation of Lao She's comment
Eunuch Pang	40 years old	male	eunuch	rich, wants a wife	–	–
Tang the Oracle	around 30 years old	male	fortune-teller	opium addict	嘴是资本奉是他先低三下四为吸大烟	A silken tongue is his capital. That helps him to polish the apple. He cringes before others to buy some opium for pleasure.
Erdez	in his twenties	male	imperial wrestler	bullies the weak	–	–
Song Enz and Wu Xiangz	in their twenties	male	old-fashioned secret agents	two wicked bullies	贵族爪牙就是他俩狗仗人势一点不假	They are two lackeys for the rich. To serve their masters, they always bully others.
Li San	in his thirties	male	waiter that works at Yutai Teahouse	hard-working and kind-hearted	–	–
Master Ma	in his thirties	male	bully	a bully who lives off the Christian missionaries	–	–
Tubby Huang	in his forties	male	underworld boss	hypocritical	–	–
Old man	82 years old	male	vendor of small goods	destitute	–	–
Peasant woman	in her thirties	female	mother of the little girl	tries to sell the little girl because of poverty	–	–
Little girl	10 years old	female	daughter of the peasant woman	poor and hungry	–	–
Kang Shunz	15 years old	female	daughter of Kang Liu	poor girl being sold to Eunuch Pang to be his wife	–	–

(see Example 2.4), and the declaratives tend to be translated as wh- interrogatives or imperatives to threaten Kang Liu (see Examples 2.6 and 2.7). When speaking to Master Song and Master Chang, the Manchurian customers and also his potential customers, he is kind and friendly, and even offers his watch to Master Song. Some imperatives are translated as declaratives, with modulated use of modality added to make them indirect (see Examples 2.9, 2.10, 2.11).

Wang Lifa, the manager of Yutai Teahouse, is tactful in dealing with different kinds of customers. He has interacted with many of the characters in the first act of the play. In terms of power and status roles, Kang Liu, Li San, the peasant woman, and Tang the Oracle's social statuses are lower than Wang Lifa's, because they are either bankrupted or have a relatively lower status in society compared to Wang Lifa's. For regular customers of the teahouse, including Master Chang and Master Song, their social statuses are equal to Wang Lifa's. For entrepreneurs, officers, and villains, including Master Qin, Eunuch Pang, Song Enz, Wu Xiangz, Erdez, Master Ma, and Tubby Huang, their social statuses are higher than Wang Lifa's. The mood analysis of the ST shows that Wang Lifa adopts different strategies to deal with different people in the teahouse. To people with a lower social status, such as Tang the Oracle and the little girl being sold by her mother, he uses a large number of imperatives. These clauses realize the speech function of "command," and by using these imperatives, Wang Lifa asks these people to go out of the teahouse. When interacting with Li San, most of the clauses he uses are also imperatives, with the aim of commanding him to provide goods and services to other customers. To people with a higher social status, including Qin Zhongyi, Eunuch Pang, Master Song, and Master Chang, Wang Lifa also uses imperatives, but here the speech function is "offer," i.e. to provide goods and services. Many of these imperatives function as commands, i.e. to ask these people to take a seat. This explains why a large amount of imperatives are used by Wang Lifa compared with the other characters. In the TTs, Wang Lifa's imperatives addressed to those either with higher or lower statuses are often translated as other mood types, such as wh- interrogatives and declaratives (see Examples 2.13–2.18). Thus, the translators tend not to translate Wang Lifa's commands directly in the TTs.

Master Chang is upright and honest. Compared to Song Enz and Wu Xiangz, the two secret agents that work for the imperial court, Master Chang has a lower status, but he is unyielding. In the ST, various declaratives are addressed to Master Song while discussing state affairs or showing his concern for the empire. Most imperatives are addressed to Erdez, Li San, and the two secret agents. In this way, he challenges Erdez over Erdez's impotence in fighting with the foreigners, he orders the bowls of noodles for the poor girl by addressing Li San, and he declines the two secret agents' request to chain him while being arrested. Interrogatives are either used to question Erdez before starting their fight, or to ask the two secret agents about the law case he is involved in. In the TTs, the interrogatives and imperatives addressed to Erdez, Song Enz, and Wu Xiangz in the ST tend to be translated as other mood types, especially in TT1 (see Examples 2.20–2.22) to question the addressees directly or to infuriate Erdez to start a fight. Master Chang's status is equal to his friend, Master Song, and is higher than the assistant of the teahouse, Li San. It is also found that one imperative addressed to Master Song in the ST is translated as declarative and yes/no interrogative in the two TTs respectively (see Example 2.19).

Qin Zhongyi is rich and arrogant. His status is higher than Wang Lifa's because the housing estate of the teahouse belongs to him. His status is equal to that of Eunuch Pang, as they are both powerful and rich. In the ST, his declaratives are addressed to Wang Lifa to talk about the house, to express his idea of increasing the house rent, to state his opinions about taking back the teahouse, and to explain his plans of building a factory. When talking to Eunuch Pang, he uses declaratives only to greet him. In the TTs, shifts of mood type are especially found in the lines addressed to Wang Lifa, while those addressed to Eunuch Pang are translated equivalently. Such changes include translation shifts from imperative to declarative (see Examples 2.24 and 2.25) in both TTs, and shifts from minor to imperative in TT1 (see Example 2.26), with the aim of threatening Wang Lifa that the teahouse would be taken back.

Kang Liu's social status is lower than that of Pock-Mark Liu and Eunuch Pang. As a poor peasant, he has to choose either being starved to death or selling his daughter. When speaking to his daughter, his status is higher, as he is the father of the young girl and can decide her destiny. In the ST, Kang Liu addresses all his declaratives to Pock-Mark Liu and his daughter Kang Shunz. When talking to Pock-Mark Liu, Kang Liu uses declaratives to negotiate the issues about the business and later to explain why Shunz fainted. For the declaratives addressed to Kang Shunz, they are either used to apologize for selling her or to explain the reason for sending her away. Moreover, the interrogatives in the ST are all addressed to Pock-Mark Liu to discuss the price of the girl and to inquire about the person that she is being sold to. In the ST, Kang Liu contributes the smallest amount of imperatives – only one imperative is found (see Example 2.27), which is addressed to Kang Shunz to ask her to accept her miserable fate. In the TTs, especially in TT1, there are some examples of interrogatives and imperatives translated as declaratives in TT1 (see Example 2.28), with the aim of stating Kang Liu's difficult situation in a more direct way.

Master Song's status is equal to Master Chang and Pock-Mark Liu's. However, his status is lower than that of Song Enz, Wu Xiangz, Tubby Huang, and Erdez. As they are aggressive, he speaks to them indirectly. In the ST, most of his imperatives are addressed to Tubby Huang, who is a gang boss, inviting him to say a few kind words to the two secret agents. In addition, his interrogatives are used to inquire about the turbulence at the backyard, the job of Erdez, the income that Pock-Mark Liu can get by selling a girl, and the reason for the fight in the inner courtyard. In the TTs, polar interrogatives in the ST are often translated as declaratives in TT1 to recreate the casual conversation between Master Song and his friends (see Examples 2.31 and 2.32). Moodtags or interjections like "eh" are also added in TT1 to translate the speech function of "question" in the ST (see Example 2.33).

Eunuch Pang's social status is higher than the status of most characters he interacts with in the play, including Pock-Mark Liu, Kang Liu, Tubby Huang, Song Enz, and Wu Xiangz. When Master Qin talks to him in a casual manner, he becomes annoyed and submits that times have changed, as the power of the imperial court has become weaker. In the ST, the mood analysis shows that Eunuch Pang uses declaratives to comment on state affairs as well as on Qin's business. Pang uses interrogatives to ask where Pock-Mark Liu is and to negotiate the price of Kang Shunz. Besides, three rhetorical questions are found, which all realize statements and are polar interrogatives of the type. Despite Pang's high status, only three imperatives are found, which are used to assure Tang the Oracle and to invite Tubby Huang to the wedding. In the TTs, both translators prefer to translate imperatives and polar interrogatives as declaratives (see Examples 2.34, 2.35, and 2.36). In these instances, moodtags are often added to invite the addressees to give their responses.

Tang the Oracle's status is lower than that of the characters he talks to, including Wang Lifa, Qin Zhongyi, and Eunuch Pang. He begs Wang Lifa to stay in the teahouse so that he can earn some money to buy opium by telling the customers' fortunes. In the ST, only declaratives and imperatives are found, while no interrogative clause is seen. These declaratives are used to ask for a cup of tea, to try to find a customer, or to give an excuse for staying in the teahouse. All three imperatives are addressed to Wang Lifa, with the aim of asking the manager of the teahouse to serve him some tea. In the TTs, imperatives of the oblative subtype are often translated as declaratives, with the speech function of "offer" remaining unchanged (see Example 2.37).

Erdez is an imperial wrestler who is invited to the teahouse to join a fight and settle a dispute at the backyard. His status is equal to that of Master Chang, who is unyielding in front of him. However, his status is obviously lower than that of Master Ma, who is another thug that scolds him and stops him from fighting, for the reason that Master Ma knows foreigners and can get help from them. In the ST, a large number of Erdez's interrogatives are used to challenge and threaten Master Chang. He also uses declaratives and one interrogative to greet Master Ma and to promise to pay for Master Ma's tea. In the TTs, some mood shifts with a limited frequency are found, such as imperative to minor (Example 2.40), elemental interrogative to declarative (Example 2.41), and polar interrogative to declarative (Example 2.42).

The status of Song Enz and Wu Xiangz's is higher than most characters', because they have the power to arrest almost everyone they dislike. However, their status is lower than that of Eunuch Pang; thus, they have to be obedient to Eunuch Pang and greet him politely. In the ST, a large proportion of the clauses they contributed are interrogatives and imperatives. These clauses have congruently realized the speech functions of "question" and "command," which help Lao She to create a terrifying atmosphere in the teahouse as well as in the Late-Qing era. In the TTs, polar interrogatives tend to be translated as declaratives, with moodtags sometimes being added (see Examples 2.42 and 2.43).

As the assistant of the teahouse, Li San's status is lower than most characters', including his boss Wang Lifa and various customers such as Master Chang and Master Song. However, compared to the social status of Kang Liu, the old man, and the peasant woman, the status of Li San is higher. He is kind to the poor people and often gives tea to them. In the ST, Li San's declaratives are mostly used to discuss the fight in the inner courtyard, and his imperatives are used to drive the old man and the little girl outside, to provide noodles to the little girl, and to advise Master Song to stop commenting on the fight. One interrogative is only used to inquire about the old man's age. In the TTs, his imperatives and wh- interrogatives tend to be translated as declaratives (see Examples 2.46, 2.47, 2.48), a pattern similar to how Wang Lifa's lines are translated throughout the play.

5.2.3   Mode of dramatic dialogue

The mode of dramatic dialogue has been described as follows.

First, the rhetorical mode of the dramatic dialogue in the ST and both TTs is dramatizing and entertaining, rather than essayistic, exploratory, didactic, explanatory, exhortatory, etc. However, by watching or reading *Teahouse*, audiences or readers can also witness the social changes brought by the three different historical eras based on their own understanding of the plot.

Second, the medium of the ST and TT2 is written to be spoken and to be performed aloud, as the primary concern for Lao She and Ying Ruocheng is to put the play on stage (Ying 1999; Ying & Conceison 2009). We can also associate this with the use of colloquial language in the ST and TT2. However, TT1, translated by John Howard-Gibbon, is written to be read, as the translator was not concerned about performability during his process of translating the play (Howard-Gibbon 2004; cf. Ren 2008).

Third, the channel of the ST is written and phonic, as the ST has been printed out in book copies and put on stage by Beijing People's Art Theatre. The channel of both TTs is the written mode, as they are published as books and used as subtitles for drama performances. TT1 has been used as subtitles in the performance in Exposition 1986 in Vancouver and an off-Broadway production by the Pan-Asian Repertory Theatre staged in New York (Howard-Gibbon 2004), while TT2 has been used as subtitles by the Beijing People's Art Theatre for its various performances in various English-speaking countries and regions since the 1980s.

Fourth, the orientation of the ST and the TTs is field-oriented, as plot plays a key role in drama.

Fifth, in terms of turn-ranking, the ST and the TTs are dialogic, as the data of dramatic dialogue in *Teahouse* is composed of dialogues only.

These descriptions of mode are suitable to be related to the analysis of Theme (see Wang 2017). Based on the differences in terms of medium and channel, we can see that the two translators (especially the translator of TT2) have adopted different strategies in order to recreate a dramatizing text to be spoken or performed on stage. Wang (2017) has made the following observations. First, the choices of recreating conversations in the ST are generally adopted by both translators, and similar frequencies of Theme shift are found in both TTs. Second, the translator of TT2 has increased a large number of continuatives that function as textual Themes, which help to start new moves in the conversations and are capable of drawing the attention of the audience. Though both translators attempt to use such continuatives, the frequency is higher in TT2 than in TT1 (see Table 3.2).

5.3 Contextual analysis of dramatic monologue

5.3.1 Field of dramatic monologue

The field of activity recreated in the dramatic monologue include exploring, reporting, and recommending. Before each act of the play, the story-teller in the dramatic monologue, i.e. Silly Young, expresses his stance by way of chanting rhythmic storytelling. The purpose of creating this character is to introduce the various situations in the teahouse (see e.g. Jiao 2007; Zhang 2008), such as what people do in the teahouse, how the manager renovates the teahouse, and how helpless the manager eventually becomes. Also, the historical background of the different eras is reported, such as the reform campaign in the Qing Dynasty, the fights between warlords during the Republican period, and the Japanese occupation. Additionally, there is the recommending field of activity, as the character tries to fulfil his own job, i.e. to beg money from other people, leading to the doing activity.

In the two TTs, the field of activity remains unchanged. Despite the large number of Theme shifts analyzed in Chapter 3 (see Table 3.6), the clauses that are used to introduce the teahouse, to comment on the historical background of the eras, and to beg for money have all been retained. A transitivity analysis in the pilot study revealed that despite the omissions and additions found in the data of dramatic monologue, many of the process types in the ST have been translated equivalently in both TTs.

5.3.2 Tenor of dramatic monologue

The tenor relation between the writer/translators and the audience is the same as previously discussed in Section 5.2.2.1. Therefore, only the relationships between the character in the play and the audience will be analyzed here. In terms of institutional role, Silly Young is a beggar chanting rhythmic storytelling in the teahouse, and he is the only character in the dramatic monologue. Compared to the other characters in the play, he has less power due to his institutional role. In addition, he and the audience are distant from each other. Before he introduces himself to the audience, they are complete strangers. His evaluation of the state affairs is thus presented from his personal point of view.

In terms of lexicogrammar, the mood analysis in the ST conducted in the pilot study showed that most of the clauses are declarative and bound clauses, as the dramatic monologue is written for introductory purposes. In the TTs, these clauses are mostly equivalently translated. In contrast to the dramatic dialogue analyzed in Chapter 2, changes in mood types are not frequently found.

5.3.3 Mode of dramatic monologue

The rhetorical mode, channel, and orientation between the ST and both TTs are the same as those previously analyzed in Section 5.2.3. Some observations are made in terms of medium and turn-ranking. The ST of dramatic monologue is written to be spoken and is monologic. It is composed in the form of Chinese rhythmic storytelling, which used to be the beggars' means of making a living and is now considered as a kind of artistic form. The language of rhythmic storytelling is concise. The lines are written in couplets, with end rhymes used at the end of each line. For the two TTs, TT1 is written to be read, while TT2 is translated into colloquial and simple language, with the aim of being performed (Ying 1999). In addition, based on the recollections of an actor in this play and an interpreter for the performances in Western Europe, it is believed that the use of colloquial language is closely related to the stage effect in performance (Gu 2010; Huo 1983; cf. Wang & Ma 2016).

We can relate the lexicogrammatical analysis in Chapter 3 to the contextual descriptions of mode in two respects. First, more conjunctions functioning as textual Themes are added in TT1 rather than TT2 (see Table 3.2), indicating that the translator of TT1 has attempted to equivalently recreate the logico-semantic relations and to mark such relations out explicitly in his translation. This is because TT1 is written to be read rather than spoken. Second, more marked topical Themes and circumstances functioning as topical Themes are found in TT2 (see Tables 3.4 and 3.5, and Examples 3.10, 3.12, 3.26). The frequencies are higher in TT2 than in TT1, as circumstances and Complements are often given thematic position in TT2 when the translator puts other elements in culminative position so as to rhyme in every two lines. Third, in general, the frequency of Theme shift is higher in TT2 than in TT1 (see Table 3.6). The occurrences of the three categories of Theme shift, i.e. Theme addition, Theme omission, and Theme substitution, are also higher in TT2 than in TT1. It is suggested that to recreate the rhythmic storytelling suitable for chanting, the translator of TT2 has made various inequivalent Theme choices in the ST.

5.4 Contextual analysis of stage direction

5.4.1 Field of stage direction

The fields of reporting and enabling are recreated in the stage direction of *Teahouse*. Specifically, in the data of stage direction, the playwright has reported: (i) the functions of the teahouse, (ii) the importance of the teahouse, (iii) the method of stage design in the three acts, and (iv) the characters onstage at the beginning of the three acts. In addition, the stage direction enables and instructs directors and actors to perform the play, leading to doing activities in real life.

In Figure 5.2, the logico-semantic (rhetorical) structure of the stage direction at the beginning of Act One is mapped out by using Rhetorical Structure Theory (RST) (e.g. Mann, Matthiessen & Thompson 1992; Matthiessen 2002). The nucleus-satellite relation links the beginning of stage direction, for example "幕启" (PY: mù qǐ; IG: curtain rise) in the ST, "The curtain rises" in TT2, with the main body of the stage direction by using the logical relation of circumstance. The multi-nuclear relations indicate that the four different parts of the text are of equal status. We can see that in the ST and both TTs, all segments of the ST are translated in

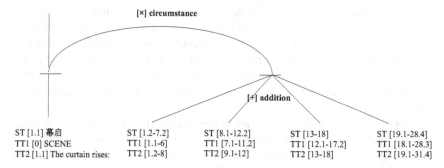

Figure 5.2 Logico-semantic (rhetorical) structure of the stage direction in Act One

the TTs, while no omission is made in the TTs. A transitivity analysis in the pilot study also suggests that the process types in the ST are mostly construed equivalently. Equivalents rather than shifts are found from this perspective.

Though experiences are reconstrued equivalently in the TTs, our lexicogrammatical analysis has pointed out the different choices made by the playwright and the two translators in systems of TAXIS and LOGICO-SEMANTIC TYPE. For instance, the playwright and the two translators have different styles in choosing tactic relations, as parataxis is preferred in the ST and hypotaxis is frequently selected in TT2. Also, we find that the preferred logico-semantic type of extension (+) in the ST has seldom been equivalently reconstrued in both TTs, with omissions of such relations frequently found (see Example 4.8).

5.4.2 Tenor of stage direction

Because stage direction is written to be read rather than to be performed, there is only the relationship between playwright/translators and readers. As we previously pointed out in Chapter 4, the readers of stage direction are likely to be professionals such as directors and actors who try to perform the play on stage and readers who appreciate the playscript as a piece of literary work. Compared to the readers, the playwright/translators are authorities. While the readers are unseen and unknown, the playwright/translators are unfamiliar with the readers, and their power relations are unequal.

In terms of lexicogrammar, the mood types of the clauses in the ST are mostly declaratives and bound clauses, as stage direction mainly serves descriptive purposes, i.e. to describe how the stage should be set and what the characters should look like. When being translated, these mood types are equivalently reenacted in the TTs.

5.4.3 Mode of stage direction

We find some common features in terms of mode in stage direction between the ST and TTs.

First, the rhetorical mode of stage direction adds some extra information about performance that is not stated in the dramatic dialogue and dramatic monologue, such as directions about stage design and descriptions of the characters' personality (cf. Hartnoll & Found 1996). Second, the medium of stage direction is written to be read by readers rather than written to be spoken or performed. Third, the channel is written words only, as this type of text will not be read aloud on stage. Fourth, in terms of turn-ranking, stage direction is monologic rather than dialogic.

These contextual descriptions of mode can be related to the lexicogrammatical analysis (see Wang 2017). As the two TTs share the same contextual features, such as those of rhetorical mode, medium, channel, and turn-ranking, similarities rather than differences are found between the TTs. The following observations about the differences are made based on the analysis: (i) Since stage direction is translated to be read, both translators tend to omit the logico-semantic relations in the ST, and they often combine several clauses in the ST to one clause in the TTs (see Examples 4.5 and 4.10). (ii) Both translators tend to reconstrue paratactically related clauses or several independent clauses in the ST to hypotactically related ones, leading to additions of hypotaxis and alterations from parataxis to hypotaxis (see Table 4.13, Examples 4.14 and 4.15). (iii) Conjunctions functioning as textual Themes are added to both TTs. This is also one of the major type of Theme shifts in terms of quantitative distribution (see Wang 2017). The conjunctions added include "and," "then," "before," "after," and "or," which change the implicit logico-semantic relations in the ST to explicitly and cohesively related clauses.

6 Conclusion

Toward a systemic functional account of drama translation

In this chapter, we first synthesize the major findings from Chapter 2 to Chapter 5 in accordance with the analytical framework proposed in Chapter 1. Then, in Section 6.2, we highlight the contributions of this study in terms of the appliability of SFL theory, the development of "the environments of translation" and "metafunctional translation shift" proposed by Matthiessen (2001, 2014b), the validity of the analytical framework proposed, the implications for translation practice and typological studies, and the investigations on translation universals. In Section 6.3, we recommend some directions for future research.

6.1 Application of the theoretical framework in this book

This book applies SFL to study drama translation by analyzing the playscript of *Teahouse* written in Chinese and its two English translations. In the playscript, three kinds of text are found, i.e. dramatic dialogue, dramatic monologue, and stage direction. Based on a pilot study, we have built a theoretical framework for the analysis that identifies choices made in the three kinds of text. In dramatic dialogue, choices in the system of MOOD are analyzed and compared. In dramatic monologue, choices in THEME are investigated. In stage direction, choices in TAXIS and LOGICO-SEMANTIC TYPE are examined. Various kinds of metafunctional translation shifts are then identified, quantified, and discussed based on the matrix of metafunctional translation shifts proposed in Matthiessen (2014b). It is found that both translators have to shift in one dimension or two to gain equivalence elsewhere, as equivalence cannot be maintained at all levels and in all dimensions. Taken together, the selected systemic analyses have offered a revealing account of how the discourse of *Teahouse* is organized to effectively function in its context of situation as well as context of culture.

In Chapter 2, we conduct the mood analysis in the dramatic dialogue of *Teahouse*. The identified mood types are related to the characterization of the play, as different mood types are helpful in understanding the creation and recreation of the characters. Some patterns in both TTs are found. For instance, among Pock-Mark Liu's clauses addressed to Kang Liu – the poor peasant forced to sell his daughter – interrogatives tend to be translated as declaratives to add more certainty to Pock-Mark Liu's assertions, and declaratives tend to be translated as wh- interrogatives or imperatives to urge Kang Liu to quickly make up his mind in selling his daughter, as Pock-Mark Liu is both created and recreated as a cruel and remorseless human trafficker.

In Chapter 3, we analyze the dramatic monologue of *Teahouse* from the perspective of Theme. The analysis reveals that a large amount of textual Themes are found in the TTs. There is no equivalent choice of textual Theme translated from the ST, and most textual Themes in the TTs are conjunctions added by the translators. A slight increase in interpersonal Themes is found in the TTs, especially in TT2, and the added interpersonal Themes are mostly Finite verbal operators. In TT2, modal/comment Adjuncts and Vocatives are also added as interpersonal Themes. For topical Themes, a much larger number of them are found in the TTs, especially in TT2, as the translator of TT2 has deliberately selected circumstances and Complements as marked topical Themes to rhyme the couplets. Additionally, fewer participants as topical Themes are found in the TTs, compared to the frequency in the ST, because both translators tend to combine the clauses in the ST that are similar in structure.

In Chapter 4, we analyze the stage direction of *Teahouse* from the perspectives of taxis and logico-semantic type. In terms of taxis, parataxis is the preferred choice in the ST, and hypotaxis is the preferred choice in TT2. For TT1, the choices of parataxis and hypotaxis are similar in frequency. For logico-semantic type, the dominant choice is that of expansion, while choices of projection are rarely found in the TTs. The preferred choice of logico-semantic type in the ST is extension, which is seldom translated equivalently in the TTs.

In Chapter 5, after the lexicogrammatical analysis, the contexts of the ST and the two TTs are described and compared in accordance with the three contextual parameters, i.e. field, tenor, and mode. The contextual analysis is further related to the translators' lexicogrammatical choices. The analysis of Theme reveals the mode of the discourse, giving an indication of how the discourse is organized and planned. The features of mood and speech function are related to the tenor and the interpersonal relations in the discourse. The analysis of taxis and logico-semantic type help us identify how spoken and written mode in the text is constructed as well as the field of discourse.

Some similarities and differences between the ST and the TTs are discussed. In the analysis of field, though the primary field of activity is recreating, the activities being recreated in different texts are summarized according to the primary eight types. The fields of activity being recreated in dramatic dialogue include exploring, recommending, enabling, sharing, and doing; the fields in dramatic monologue include exploring, reporting, and recommending; and the fields in stage direction are reporting and enabling. It is found that the fields in the three types of text are all recreated equivalently. The description of tenor in dramatic dialogue and dramatic monologue are analyzed in a two-fold way, consisting of the tenor relations between writer/translators and readers as well as those between the various characters in the play. Some differences are summarized in terms of institutional role, power and status roles, and distance. The analysis of mode is carried out from the perspectives of rhetorical mode, medium, channel, orientation, and turn-ranking.

A significant difference observed is that the ST and TT2 are written to be spoken and to be performed aloud, as a result of Lao She's concern of staging the play in Beijing People's Art Theatre in the year of 1958 as well as Ying Ruocheng's consideration of performability in his translation. However, John-Howard Gibbon's translation is written to be read; thus, performability is not considered during his process of translation (Howard-Gibbon 2004).

The contextual analysis provides evidence for the lexicogrammatical choices discussed from Chapter 2 to Chapter 4, as the translators' choices are to some extent influenced by the context. To take dramatic monologue as an example, quantitatively speaking, TT1 is much closer to the ST than TT2 in many respects, such as the use of interpersonal Theme, marked topical Theme, and unmarked topical Theme. As TT1 is translated to be read rather than performed, it has a lower requirement for rhyme scheme or the use of colloquial language. From the analysis of tenor and mode, we can see that in order to realize the performability of the translation, Ying Ruocheng, the translator of TT2, has to make various changes to the ST, such as increasing the use of marked topical Theme and textual Theme.

The framework in this book offers one empirical attempt to identify, compare, and analyze the translators' choices with the help of SFL. It is also one approach to quantitatively describe drama translation as well as the styles of the two translators. The framework is adjustable according to the texts to be selected. We can modify the systems selected in accordance with the nature of the data, the purpose of the research, etc.

6.2   Significance of the study

First, in terms of the general theory of SFL and translation studies, this book makes a theoretical contribution in its application of SFL to translation studies, specifically to the study of drama translation. Although other approaches of engaging with translation can be found in the literature (cf. Pym 2010; Gentzler 2001; Munday 2016), translation is here considered and illuminated as a linguistic process. Following this approach, the appliability of SFL is emphasized. SFL, on the other hand, as a general and holistic theory of language, is suitable to shed light on translation (see Section 1.1; Wang & Ma in press). It not only offers its accounts on language as potential, language as process, and language as instance but is also a meaning-oriented theory, thus making it possible to see how the different modes of meaning are construed, enacted, organized, or balanced in text. More importantly, in SFL, language is studied in relation to context, with an orientation toward the paradigmatic axis. Therefore, the language of the data in the present study, i.e. dramatic text, is considered here as resources that are organized as choices chosen by the playwright and the two translators in the meaning potential of the source language and the target language.

SFL has always taken translation seriously by considering translation as part of linguistic theory (Matthiessen, Wang & Ma 2017a, 2017b, 2018). Such a theory provides answers to the two questions Firth (1968a: 83) raised, i.e. "Do we know how we translate?" and "Do we even know what we translate?" when he emphasizes the need to study translation from a linguistic perspective (cf. Firth 1968b). It is against this backdrop that we have selected SFL as the theory to analyze and compare the choices in the ST and the two TTs.

Second, by integrating the dimensions outlined in Matthiessen (2001), such as stratification, metafunction, instantiation, and rank, an analytical framework is built with the purpose of applying SFL to study drama translation. In terms of stratification, our analysis starts from the lexicogrammar stratum and extends to the strata of semantics and context. In terms of rank, the lexicogrammatical analysis is carried out on clause rank, where translation shifts are examined. In terms of instantiation, the present study proceeds from the instance pole of the cline and moves toward the system pole of the cline.

Such a framework not only provides linguistic evidence to support translation evaluation and criticism (cf. House 1977, 1997, 2015) but also enables us to examine drama translation from the perspective of SFL. Modifications can be made to the framework according to the features of the text to be examined – for example, by taking other modes of meaning and other systems into consideration (cf. Ma 2018). Theoretically, this framework will be suitable for the analysis of different kinds of texts, especially drama texts or texts characterized by exchanges and dialogues. Moreover, this study is one of the first attempts to analyze Chinese drama and its translations from a systemic functional perspective.

Third, the theoretical framework is one of the first attempts to apply and further develop the notion of metafunctional translation shift proposed in Matthiessen (2014b). Based on the lexicogrammatical analysis from Chapter 2 to Chapter 5, different kinds of metafunctional translation shifts are discussed and illustrated, including Theme shift, mood shift, tactic shift, and logico-semantic type shift. These shifts are further categorized, and the more delicate subcategories are discussed.

It also becomes evident that as we explore the translation shift empirically, we can find which shifts are more likely to occur and which shifts can be found more often in which kind of data in terms of probability (e.g. the mood shifts that are related to different characters, as analyzed from Sections 2.2.2 to 2.2.12) (cf. Halliday 1991b, 1993; Toury 2004). The shifts, on the other hand, can further inform us about the different metafunctional modes of meaning and how the modes of meaning are balanced in a text.

In Matthiessen (2014b), the different kinds of metafunctional translation shifts are presented in the form of a matrix (see Figure 1.5). In this study, we observe that some boxes in the matrix are empty because such shifts have not yet been exemplified (see discussions in Matthiessen, Wang & Ma 2017a). As we further explore, analyze, and compare more translated texts with their originals, we can find other shifts between different languages, thereby helping fill in some of the boxes and finding out which boxes are likely to remain empty.

Fourth, by analyzing the data in English and Chinese, this study reflects the systemic contrasts between the two languages (e.g. differences in choices of textual Theme, in mood choices like polar interrogatives, and in logical choices of hypotactic elaboration) and contributes to multilingual studies in SFL, which include studies on language description and language typology (see Sections 2.4, 3.4, and 4.4). In addition, the detailed lexicogrammatical analysis holds implications for translation practice. Like other studies that investigate translation from an SFL perspective, the present study provides translators with the tools that can help them examine and diagnose the issues in translation. It reveals the options and challenges that translators may come across in translation (e.g. addition of certain textual Themes, awareness of differences between the two languages in terms of mood type) and provides them with additional theoretical and professional insights about language. It also helps them to be aware of the systemic probabilities, as translators are subconsciously aware of the systemic probabilities, either in terms of the general system or the generic subsystem of their translated work (cf. Catford 1965; Jesus & Pagano 2006; Matthiessen 2014b; Toury 2004).

Fifth, based on the findings of the detailed lexicogrammatical analysis carried out from Chapter 2 to Chapter 4, the present study represents a preliminary attempt to refute the claims of the existence of translation universals found in various literature on translation studies (e.g. Blum-Kulka 1986; Baker 1993; Mauranen & Kujamäki 2004; Malmkjær 2005; Mauranen 2008). According to House (2008: 10), these so-called translation universals are "universal tendencies of the translation process, laws of translation and norms of translation," which include processes, procedures or operations such as explicitation, simplification, standardization, disambiguation, levelling out, avoidance of repetition, and conventionalization, as well as the general manifestation of a "third code." Our study provides evidence for House's (2008, 2018) claim that it is futile to look for translation universals.

For instance, House (2008) confirms that linguistic theories can help us find universals of language. As translation is primarily a linguistic act, these universals can certainly be applied to translation. However, these are not universals of translation per se but rather universals of language being applied to translation. This book adopts SFL as its theoretical basis and has successfully discovered some typological features that operate both in Chinese and English, such as similarities in the basic choices in the systems of THEME, MOOD, TAXIS, and LOGICO-SEMANTIC TYPE and similarities in the elements that function as marked topical Themes. More linguistic analyses between the two languages will identify more of such shared features and apply such findings to translation. Whether these features are universals or not will then depend on further studies on an even larger number of languages.

Also, House (2008) locates acts of translation at the instance pole of the cline of instantiation, i.e. as acts of performance or parole, and emphasizes that translation is dependent on the language pair involved. Given the large number of languages spoken around the world, the translation universals found in some language pairs may not work in some other pairs (see Grace 1981; Pawley 1987). Therefore, claims like "explicitation" should be made under solid and linguistic scrutiny (e.g. Hansen-Schirra, Neumann & Steiner 2012). In the present study, some shifts can make the translations more explicit, such as shifts from textual to logical (see Example 3.2) and the addition of conjunctions as textual Themes (see Example 3.14), but these explicitations are due to typological differences rather than the existence of translation universals. Moreover, some shifts can make the translations more implicit, such as the omission of conjunction as textual Theme (see Example 3.20) and the omission of topical Theme (see Example 3.22).

Further, House (2008) draws our attention to the issue of directionality, which is closely related to language-pair specificity. For instance, some procedures of explicitation found in translations from Chinese to English will not work in the opposite direction, i.e. in translations from English to Chinese. In the case of this book, if we translate the dramatic dialogue and dramatic monologue back from English to Chinese, many of the conjunctions that function as textual Themes in English will have to be left out and translated implicitly in the Chinese translation. On the one hand, fewer conjunctions are found in Chinese, in accordance with various studies on language description and typology (e.g. Chao 1968; Li & Thompson 1981; Li 2007). On the other hand, as the registers of the data are daily conversation and rhythmic storytelling, which are written to be spoken and chanted, conjunctions in Chinese will be redundant (see Example 3.2).

In addition, House (2008) takes the universals in translation as genre specific. In some texts, some tendencies of certain universals will be found, while in others, the situation will be different. In the present study, three kinds of text are involved in the analysis, i.e. dramatic dialogue, dramatic monologue, and stage direction. Shifts of mood type are only frequently found in the data of dramatic dialogue, with various examples of substituting one mood type with another being observed (see Section 2.3). However, in the data of dramatic monologue and stage direction, mood choices remain equivalent in general, as most of the clauses are declaratives and are often translated equivalently. It is also for this reason that the system of MOOD is excluded for the analysis of stage direction and dramatic monologue in this book.

6.3   Some thoughts for future work

There are some limitations of the present study, despite its contributions to the scholarship on translation.

First, the data of dramatic dialogue and stage direction are relatively small, especially those of the stage direction, which only consist of the beginning part of the descriptions of stage setting and character introduction, because a large part of the English translation of stage direction is composed of non-Finite clauses. More findings are likely to be revealed if a larger sample of texts are collected and analyzed; this will enable a profile of probability to be built.

Second, based on our pilot study, some systems in some modes of meaning are not considered in the lexicogrammatical analysis, such as TRANSITIVITY, MODALITY, POLARITY, and SUBJECT PERSON. Though they are not considered here in the study, they are important and worthy of investigation. If we expand our data and analyze them in terms of a larger number of systems, we can expect more findings (see e.g. Ma 2018 for transitivity analysis of poetry translation).

Third, this study only takes two English translations of *Teahouse* and the source text written in Chinese into consideration. As *Teahouse* is a highly valued and influential text in Chinese literature, it has been translated into various languages, such as German, French, Spanish, and Japanese. It should be desirable to analyze the translations in different languages, to observe the similarities and differences between the ST and the various TTs, and to promote the notion of multilingual studies emphasized in Matthiessen, Teruya, and Wu (2008) (see also Bateman, Matthiessen & Zeng 1999).

Given the limitations of the study, future work can be carried out along the following lines.

First, the whole ST and the TTs can be included in the analysis in order to construct probability profiles of choices made both in the Chinese original and in the two English translations. In addition, the different translations of *Teahouse* can be collected as data for future research (cf. Wang & Ma 2016 for possibilities of translating *Teahouse* from Mandarin Chinese to Cantonese).

Second, more studies can be carried out by analyzing other types of texts, such as poetry (e.g. Ma 2018), advertisement (e.g. Steiner 2004), legal documents (e.g. Espindola & Wang 2015), and Buddhist sutras (e.g. Yu & Wu 2016, 2017). In this way, texts from different fields of activity are analyzed in order to discuss the translation strategies across various registers and to ascertain how different sociosemiotic processes can influence the translators' strategies.

Third, we can generate more insights from the translators' editing process. If we can include Ying Ruocheng's drafts of his translation as part of the data, we can compare his draft with the published versions of *Teahouse* from an informed linguistic point of view (cf. Yang 2016).

Fourth, an interesting area of research will be the performability of drama and its relation to translation from one language to the other and vice versa. For example, we can compare Ying Ruocheng's translations of drama from Chinese to English, such as *Teahouse*, *The Family*, and *Uncle Doggie's Nirvana*, with his translations from English to Chinese, such as *Death of a Salesman*, *Major Barbara*, *The Caine Mutiny Court-Martial*, *Amadeus*, and *Measure for Measure*. Based on the SFL analysis, we can ascertain whether he uses the same strategies while translating plays from Chinese to English and from English to Chinese.

Fifth, more theoretical development of SFL is needed. SFL, as one kind of applicable linguistics, will continue to evolve in the future. It is hoped that our analysis can shed light on the theoretical development of SFL to promote a more productive and effective continuation of the theory. Instead of merely applying insights that have already been established theoretically, we hope that our study can feed back into the development of the theory.

References

Austin, J.L. 1962. *How to do things with words*. Oxford: Claredon Press.

Baker, Mona. 1992. *In other words: A coursebook in translation*. London & New York: Routledge.

Baker, Mona. 1993. "Corpus linguistics and translation studies: Implications and applications." In Mona Baker, Gill Francis & Elena Tognini-Bonelli (eds.), *Text and technology: In honour of John Sinclair*. Amsterdam & Philadelphia: John Benjamins. 233–250.

Bateman, John A., Christian M.I.M. Matthiessen & Licheng Zeng. 1999. "Multilingual language generation for multilingual software: A functional linguistic approach." *Applied Artificial Intelligence: An International Journal* 13(6): 607–639.

Bell, Roger. 1991. *Translation and translating: Theory and practice*. London & New York: Longman.

Blum-Kulka, Shoshana. 1986. "Shifts of cohesion and coherence in translation." In Juliane House & Shoshana Blum-Kulka (eds.), *Interlingual and intercultural communication: Discourse and cognition in translation and second language acquisition*. Tübingen: Gunter Narr. 17–35.

Blum-Kulka, Shoshana & Juliane House. 1989. "Cross-cultural and situational variation in requesting behaviour." In Shoshana Blum-Kulka, Juliane House & Gabriele Kasper (eds.), *Cross-cultural pragmatics: Requests and apologies*. Norwood: Ablex. 123–154.

Butt, David G., Rhondda Fahey, Susan Feez, Sue Spinks & Colin Yallop. 1994. *Using functional grammar: An explorer's guide*. Sydney: National Centre for English Language Teaching and Research.

Butt, David G. & Rebekah Kate Ardley Wegener. 2007. "The work of concepts: Context and metafunction in the systemic functional model." In Ruqaiya Hasan, Christian M.I.M. Matthiessen & Jonathan Webster (eds.), *Continuing discourse on language: A functional perspective* (volume 2). London: Equinox. 589–618.

Caffarel, Alice, James R. Martin & Christian M.I.M. Matthiessen. (eds.). 2004. *Language typology: A functional perspective*. Amsterdam & Philadelphia: John Benjamins.

Cao, Yu [曹禺]. (2007). "曹禺谈《茶馆》[Cao Yu on *Teahouse*]." In 刘章春 [Liu Zhangchun] (ed.), 《茶馆》的舞台艺术 [Arts of *Teahouse*]. 北京 [Beijing]: 中国戏剧出版社 [China Theatre Press]. 186–188.

Catford, J.C. 1965. *A linguistic theory of translation*. London: Oxford University Press.

Chao, Yuen Ren. 1968. *A grammar of spoken Chinese*. Berkeley, Los Angeles & London: University of California Press.

Chomsky, Noam. 1957. *Syntactic structures*. The Hague: Mouton.

Chomsky, Noam. 1965. *Aspects of the theory of syntax*. Cambridge: MIT Press.

Chomsky, Noam. 2006. *Language and mind*. Cambridge: Cambridge University Press.

Corder, Stephen Pit. 1967. "The significance of learners' errors." *International Review of Applied Linguistics* 5: 160–170.

Daneš, František. 1974. "Functional sentence perspective and the organization of the text." In František Daneš (ed.), *Papers on functional sentence perspective*. The Hague: Mouton. 106–128.

Espindola, Elaine & Yan Wang. 2015. "The enactment of modality in regulatory texts: A comparative study of tenancy agreements." *Journal of World Languages* 2(2–3): 106–125.

Feng, Yuanzheng [冯远征]. 2007. "蜕变 – 我演松二爷 [Metamorphosis: How do I play Master Song]." In 刘章春 [Liu Zhangchun] (ed.), 《茶馆》的舞台艺术 [Arts of *Teahouse*]. 北京 [Beijing]: 中国戏剧出版社 [China Theatre Press]. 180–183.

Firbas, Jan. 1964. "On defining the theme in functional sentence analysis." *Travaux Linguistiques de Prague* 1: 267–280.

Firbas, Jan. 1992. *Functional sentence perspective in written and spoken communication.* Cambridge & New York: Cambridge University Press.

Firth, J.R. 1957. *Papers in linguistics 1934–1951.* London: Oxford University Press.

Firth, J.R. 1968a. "Linguistic analysis and translation." In F.R. Palmer (ed.), *Selected papers of J.R. Firth 1952–59.* London & Harlow: Longmans. 74–83.

Firth, J.R. 1968b. "Linguistics and translation." In F.R. Palmer (ed.), *Selected papers of J.R. Firth 1952–59.* London & Harlow: Longmans. 84–95.

Fries, Peter H. 1981. "On the status of theme in English: Arguments from discourse." *Forum Linguisticum* 6(1): 1–38. Reprinted in J. Petöfi & E. Sözer (ed.), *Micro and macro connexity of texts*. Hamburg: Helmut Buske Verlag. 116–152.

Fries, Peter H. 1995. "A personal view of theme." In Mohsen Ghadessy (ed.), *Thematic development in English texts*. London & New York: Pinter. 1–19.

Gentzler, Edwin. 2001. *Contemporary translation theories.* Clevedon: Multilingual Matters.

Ghadessy, Mohsen. 1995. "Thematic development and its relationship to registers and genres." In Mohsen Ghadessy (ed.), *Thematic development in English texts*. London & New York: Pinter. 129–146.

Goatly, Andrew. 1995. "Marked Theme and its interpretation in A.E. Houseman's *A Shropshire Lad*." In Mohsen Ghadessy (ed.), *Thematic development in English texts*. London & New York: Pinter. 164–197.

Grace, George W. 1981. *An essay on language.* Columbia: Hornbeam Press.

Gu, Wei [顾威]. 2010. "谈人艺的艺术风格 [On the artistic style of Beijing People's Art Theatre]." In 刘章春 [Liu Zhangchun] (ed.), 人艺批评: 北京人艺戏剧理论集2002–2007 [A collection of academic theories of Beijing People's Art Theatre 2002–2007]. 北京 [Beijing]: 中国戏剧出版社 [China Theatre Press]. 112–108.

Guo, Cong [郭聪] & Weiwei Ding [丁娓娓]. 2009. "从《茶馆》的两个译本看感叹词的翻译 [The translation of interjections in the two translations of *Teahouse*]." 内蒙古农业大学学报 [Journal of Inner Mongolia Agricultural University] 11(3): 392–394.

Halliday, M.A.K. 1956. "The linguistic basis of a mechanical thesaurus, and its application to English preposition classification." *Mechanical Translation* 3: 81–88. Reprinted in M.A.K. Halliday. 2005. Jonathan J. Webster (ed.), *Computational and quantitative studies: Volume 6* in the *Collected works of M.A.K. Halliday*. London & New York: Continuum. 6–19.

Halliday, M.A.K. 1961. "Categories of the theory of grammar." *Word* 17: 241–292. Reprinted in M.A.K. Halliday. 2002. Jonathan J. Webster (ed.), *On grammar: Volume 1* in the *Collected works of M.A.K. Halliday*. London & New York: Continuum. 37–94.

Halliday, M.A.K. 1962. "Linguistics and machine translation." *Zeitschrift für Phonetik, Sprachwissenschaft und Kommunikationsforschung* 15: 145–158. Reprinted in M.A.K. Halliday. 2005. Jonathan J. Webster (ed.), *Computational and quantitative studies: Volume 6* in the *Collected works of M.A.K. Halliday*. London & New York: Continuum. 20–36.

Halliday, M.A.K. 1964. "Syntax and the consumer." In C.I.J.M. Stuart (ed.), *Report of the fifteenth annual (first international) round table meeting on linguistics and language study*. Washington, DC: Georgetown University Press. 11–24. Reprinted in M.A.K. Halliday & James R. Martin (eds.). 1981. *Readings in systemic linguistics*. London: Batsford. 21–28. Reprinted in M.A.K. Halliday. 2003. Jonathan J. Webster (ed.), *On language and linguistics: Volume 3* in the *Collected works of M.A.K. Halliday*. London & New York: Continuum. 36–49.

Halliday, M.A.K. 1967a. "Notes on transitivity and theme in English: Part I." *Journal of Linguistics* 3: 37–82. Reprinted in M.A.K. Halliday. 2005. Jonathan J. Webster (ed.), *Studies in English language: Volume 7* in the *Collected works of M.A.K. Halliday*. London & New York: Continuum. 5–54.

Halliday, M.A.K. 1967b. "Notes on transitivity and theme in English: Part II." *Journal of Linguistics* 3: 199–244. Reprinted in M.A.K. Halliday. 2005. Jonathan J. Webster (ed.), *Studies in English language: Volume 7* in the *Collected works of M.A.K. Halliday*. London & New York: Continuum. 55–109.

Halliday, M.A.K. 1970. "Language structure and language function." In John Lyons (ed.), *New horizons in linguistics*. Harmondsworth: Penguin. 140–164. Reprinted in M.A.K. Halliday. 2002. Jonathan J. Webster (ed.), *On grammar: Volume 1* in the *Collected works of M.A.K. Halliday*. London & New York: Continuum. 173–195.

Halliday, M.A.K. 1977. "Ideas about language." *Occasional Papers I*: 32–55. Reprinted in M.A.K. Halliday. 2003. Jonathan J. Webster (ed.), *On language and linguistics: Volume 3* in the *Collected works of M.A.K. Halliday*. London & New York: Continuum. 92–115.

Halliday, M.A.K. 1978. *Language as social semiotic: The social interpretation of language and meaning*. London: Edward Arnold.

Halliday, M.A.K. 1985a. *An introduction to functional grammar*. London: Edward Arnold.

Halliday, M.A.K. 1985b. "Systemic background." In James D. Benson & William S. Greaves (eds.), *Systemic perspectives on discourse (volume 1): Selected theoretical papers from the 9th International Systemic Workshop*. Norwood: Ablex. 1–15. Reprinted in M.A.K. Halliday. 2003. Jonathan J. Webster (ed.), *On language and linguistics: Volume 3* in the *Collected works of M.A.K. Halliday*. London & New York: Continuum. 185–198.

Halliday, M.A.K. 1990. "The construction of knowledge and value in the grammar of scientific discourse: With reference to Charles Darwin's *The origin of species*." In Clotilde de Stasio, Maurizio Gotti & Rossana Bonadei (eds.), *La rappresentazione verbale e iconica: valori estetici e funzionali*. Milan: Guerini Studio. 57–80. Reprinted in M.A.K. Halliday. 2002. Jonathan J. Webster (ed.), *Linguistic studies of text and discourse: Volume 2* in the *Collected works of M.A.K. Halliday*. London & New York: Continuum. 168–192.

Halliday, M.A.K. 1991a. "The notion of 'context' in language education." In Thao Lê & Mike McCausland (eds.), *Language education: Interaction and development: Proceedings of the international conference, Vietnam, 30 March–1 April 1991*. Launceston: University of Tasmania. 1–26. Reprinted in M.A.K. Halliday. 2007. Jonathan J. Webster (ed.), *Language and education: Volume 9* in the *Collected works of M.A.K. Halliday*. London & New York: Continuum. 269–290.

Halliday, M.A.K. 1991b. "Towards probabilistic interpretations." In Eija Ventola (ed.), *Functional and systemic linguistics: Approaches and uses*. Berlin & New York: Mouton de Gruyter. 39–61. Reprinted in M.A.K. Halliday. 2005. Jonathan J. Webster (ed.), *Computational and quantitative studies: Volume 6* in the *Collected works of M.A.K. Halliday*. London & New York: Continuum. 42–62.

Halliday, M.A.K. 1993. "Quantitative studies and probabilities in grammar." In Michael Hoey (ed.), *Data, description, discourse: Papers on English language in honour of John McH. Sinclair on his sixtieth birthday*. London: Harper Collins. 1–25. Reprinted in M.A.K. Halliday. 2005. Jonathan J. Webster (ed.), *Computational and quantitative studies: Volume 6* in the *Collected works of M.A.K. Halliday*. London & New York: Continuum. 130–156.

Halliday, M.A.K. 1994a. *An introduction to functional grammar*. 2nd edition. London: Edward Arnold.

Halliday, M.A.K. 1994b. "So you say 'pass'. . . thank you three muchly." In Allen D. Grimshaw, Peter J. Burke, Aaron V. Cicourel, Jenny Cook-Gumperz, Steven Feld, Charles J. Fillmore, Lily Wong Fillmore, John J. Gumperz, Michael A.K. Halliday, Ruqaiya Hasan & David Jenness, *What's going on here? Complementary studies of professional talk (volume two of the multiple analysis project)*. Norwood: Ablex. 175–229.

Halliday, M.A.K. 1996. "On grammar and grammatics." In Ruqaiya Hasan, Carmel Cloran & David Butt (eds.), *Functional descriptions: Theory into practice*. Amsterdam: John Benjamins. 1–38. Reprinted in M.A.K. Halliday. 2002. Jonathan J. Webster (ed.), *On grammar: Volume 1* in the *Collected works of M.A.K. Halliday*. London & New York: Continuum. 384–417.

Halliday, M.A.K. 2001. "Towards a theory of good translation." In Erich Steiner & Colin Yallop (eds.), *Exploring translation and multilingual text production: Beyond content*. Berlin: Mouton de Gruyter. 13–18.

Halliday, M.A.K. 2008. "Working with meaning: Towards an appliable linguistics." In Jonathan J. Webster (ed.), *Meaning in context: Implementing intelligent applications of language studies*. London & New York: Continuum. 7–23.

Halliday, M.A.K. 2009. "The gloosy ganoderm: Systemic functional linguistics and translation." *Chinese Translators Journal* [中国翻译] 1: 17–26. Reprinted in M.A.K. Halliday. 2013. Jonathan J. Webster (ed.), *Halliday in the 21st century: Volume 11* in the *Collected works of M.A.K. Halliday*. London & New York: Bloomsbury. 105–126.

Halliday, M.A.K. 2010. "Pinpointing the choice: Meaning and the search for equivalents in a translated text." In Ahmar Mahboob & Naomi K. Knight (eds.), *Appliable linguistics*. London & New York: Continuum. 13–24. Reprinted in M.A.K. Halliday. 2013. Jonathan J. Webster (ed.), *Halliday in the 21st century: Volume 11* in the *Collected works of M.A.K. Halliday*. London & New York: Bloomsbury. 143–154.

Halliday, M.A.K. & Ruqaiya Hasan. 1976. *Cohesion in English*. London: Longman.

Halliday, M.A.K. & Ruqaiya Hasan. 1985. *Language, context, and text: A social semiotic perspective*. Victoria: Deakin University Press.

Halliday, M.A.K. & Christian M.I.M. Matthiessen. 2004. *An introduction to functional grammar*. 3rd edition. London: Edward Arnold.

Halliday, M.A.K. & Christian M.I.M. Matthiessen. 2014. *Halliday's introduction to functional grammar*. 4th edition. London & New York: Routledge.

Halliday, M.A.K. & Edward McDonald. 2004. "Metafunctional profile of the grammar of Chinese." In Alice Caffarel, James R. Martin & Christian M.I.M. Matthiessen (eds.), *Language typology: A functional perspective*. Amsterdam & Philadelphia: John Benjamins. 253–305.

Halliday, M.A.K., Angus McIntosh & Peter Strevens. 1964. *The linguistic sciences and language teaching*. London: Longman.

Hansen, Sandra & Silvia Hansen-Schirra. 2012. "Grammatical shifts in English-German noun phrases." In Silvia Hansen-Schirra, Stella Neumann & Erich Steiner (eds.), *Cross-linguistic corpora for the study of translations: Insights from the language pair English-German*. München: Walter de Gruyter. 133–145.

Hansen-Schirra, Silvia, Stella Neumann & Erich Steiner. (eds.). 2012. *Cross-linguistic corpora for the study of translations: Insights from the language pair English-German*. München: Mouton de Gruyter.

Hartnoll, Phyllis & Peter Found. (eds.). 1996. *The concise Oxford companion to the theatre*. 2nd edition. Oxford: Oxford University Press.

Hasan, Ruqaiya. 1985. *Linguistics, language and verbal art*. Geelong, Victoria: Deakin University Press.

Hasan, Ruqaiya. 2009. "The place of context in a systemic functional model." In M.A.K. Halliday & Jonathan J. Webster (eds.), *Continuum companion to systemic functional linguistics*. London & New York: Continuum. 166–189.

Hatim, Basil & Ian Mason. 1990. *Discourse and the translator*. London: Routledge.

House, Juliane. 1977. *A model for translation quality assessment*. Tübingen: Gunter Narr.

House, Juliane. 1996. "Contrastive discourse analysis and misunderstanding: The case of German and English." In Marlis Hellinger & Ulrich Ammon (eds.), *Contrastive socio-linguistics*. Berlin: de Gruyter. 345–361.

House, Juliane. 1997. *Translation quality assessment: A model revisited*. Tübingen: Gunter Narr.

House, Juliane. 1998. "Politeness and translation." In Leo Hickey (ed.), *The pragmatics of translation*. Clevedon: Multilingual Matters. 54–71.

House, Juliane. 2008. "Beyond intervention: Universals in translation?." *trans-kom* 1(1): 6–19.

House, Juliane. 2015. *Translation quality assessment: Past, present and future*. Oxon & New York: Routledge.

House, Juliane. 2018. *Translation: The basics*. Oxon & New York: Routledge.

Howard-Gibbon, John. 2004, February 13. "Counting your treasures [Online news]." Retrieved from www.chinadaily.com.cn/english/bjweekend/2004-02/13/content_305764.htm.

Hu, Jieqing [胡絜青]. (ed.). 1980. 老舍生活与创作自述 [Lao She's own account on life and creation]. 北京 [Beijing]: 三联书店 [Joint Publishing].

Huang, Guowen [黄国文]. 2006. 翻译研究的语言学探索 – 古诗词英译本的语言学分析 [Linguistic explorations in translation studies: Analysis of English translations of ancient Chinese poems and lyrics]. 上海 [Shanghai]: 上海外语教育出版社 [Shanghai Foreign Language Education Press].

Huang, Zongluo [黄宗洛]. 2007. "让角色在自己身上活起来 [Let the character be alive in me]." In 刘章春 [Liu Zhangchun] (ed.), 《茶馆》的舞台艺术 [Arts of *Teahouse*]. 北京 [Beijing]: 中国戏剧出版社 [China Theatre Press]. 94–99.

Huo, Yong [霍勇]. 1983. "《茶馆》导演、演员访问记 [Notes on the interview with director an actors from *Teahouse*]." In Uwe Kräuter (ed.), 东方舞台上的奇迹 – 《茶馆》在西欧 [A miracle on the oriental stage: *Teahouse* in West Europe]. 北京 [Beijing]: 文化艺术出版社 [Culture and Art Publishing House]. 153–175.

Jesus, Silvana Maria de & Adriana Silvina Pagano. 2006. Probabilistic grammar in translation. In *Proceedings of the 33rd International Functional Congress*. São Paulo, Brazil. 428–448.

Jiao, Juyin [焦菊隐]. 2007. "导演的构思 [Conceptions of the director]." In 刘章春 [Liu Zhangchun] (ed.), 《茶馆》的舞台艺术 [Arts of *Teahouse*]. 北京 [Beijing]: 中国戏剧出版社 [China Theatre Press]. 9–16.

Kennedy, Dennis. 2010. "Dialogue." In Dennis Kennedy (ed.), *The Oxford companion to theatre and performance*. Oxford: Oxford University Press. 166.

Kim, Mira & Zhi Huang. 2012. "Theme choices in translation and target readers' reactions to different Theme choices." *T & I Review* 2: 79–112.

Kim, Mira & Christian M.I.M. Matthiessen. 2015. "Ways to move forward in translation studies: A textual perspective." *Target* 27(3): 335–350.

Lan, Tianye [蓝天野]. 2007. "创造·生活·回忆 [Creation, life, and memory]." In 刘章春 [Liu Zhangchun] (ed.), 《茶馆》的舞台艺术 [Arts of *Teahouse*]. 北京 [Beijing]: 中国戏剧出版社 [China Theatre Press]. 88–93.

Lao, She [老舍]. 1980. 茶馆 [Teahouse] (John Howard-Gibbon, Trans.). 北京 [Beijing]: 外文出版社 [Foreign Languages Press].

Lao, She [老舍]. 1982. 老舍生活与创作自述 [Lao She's on his life and work]. 北京 [Beijing]: 人民文学出版社.

Lao, She [老舍]. 1999. 茶馆 [Teahouse] (Ying Ruocheng, Trans.). 北京 [Beijing]: 中国对外翻译出版公司 [China Translation and Publishing Corporation].

Lao, She [老舍]. 2003. 茶馆 [Teahouse] (Ying Ruocheng, Trans.). 台北 [Taipei]: 书林出版有限公司 [Bookman Publishing Corporation].

Lao, She [老舍]. 2004. 茶馆 [Teahouse] (John Howard-Gibbon, Trans.). 香港 [Hong Kong]: 中文大学出版社 [Chinese University Press].

Li, Charles N. & Sandra Thompson. 1981. *Mandarin Chinese: A functional reference grammar*. Berkeley, Los Angeles & London: University of California Press.

Li, Eden Sum-hung. 2007. *A systemic functional grammar of Chinese*. London & New York: Continuum.

Li, Xiang [李翔]. 2007. "词少，事多，也要演好 – 李三的创造札记 [Few lines, more duties, but good job required: Notes on creating Li San]." In 刘章春 [Liu Zhangchun] (Ed.), 《茶馆》的舞台艺术 [Arts of *Teahouse*]. 北京 [Beijing]: 中国戏剧出版社 [China Theatre Press]. 114–121.

Li, Yuan [李源]. 2007. "我怎样演二德子和小二德子 [How do I play Erdez Senior and Erdez Junior]." In 刘章春 [Liu Zhangchun] (Ed.), 《茶馆》的舞台艺术 [Arts of *Teahouse*]. 北京 [Beijing]: 中国戏剧出版社 [China Theatre Press]. 122–129.

Lian, Kuoru [连阔如]. 2012. 江湖丛谈 [Essays on the itinerant trades]. 北京 [Beijing]: 中华书局 [Zhonghua Book Company].

Liu, Zhangchun [刘章春]. (ed.). 2007. 《茶馆》的舞台艺术 [Arts of *Teahouse*]. 北京 [Beijing]: 中国戏剧出版社 [China Theatre Press].

Ma, Yuanyi. 2018. *A systemic functional perspective on Rabindranath Tagore's Stray Birds and its Chinese translations*. Doctoral thesis, the Hong Kong Polytechnic University, Hong Kong.

Mackenzie, Hector. 2011, September 16. "Farewell to an extraordinary man [Online news]." Retrieved from www.ross-shirejournal.co.uk/Features/Last-Word/Farewell-to-an-extraordinary-man-7206075.htm.

Malinowski, Branislow. 1923. "The problem of meaning in primitive languages." In C.K. Ogden & I.A. Richards (eds.), *The meaning of meaning*. London: Kegan Paul. 1–84.

Malinowski, Bronislaw. 1935. *Coral gardens and their magic: A study of the methods of tilling the soil and of agricultural rites in the Trobriand Islands: Volume 2: The language of magic and gardening*. New York: American Book Company.

Malmkjær, Kirsten. 2005. "Norms and nature in translation studies." *Synaps* 16: 13–20.

Mann, William C., Christian M.I.M. Matthiessen & Sandra A. Thompson. 1992. "Rhetorical Structure Theory and text analysis." In William C. Mann & Sandra A. Thompson (eds.), *Discourse description: Diverse linguistic analyses of a fund-raising text*. Amsterdam: John Benjamins. 39–79.

Martin, James R. 1983. "Participant identification in English, Tagalog and Kâte." *Australian Journal of Linguistics* 3(1): 45–74.

Martin, James R. 1995. "More than what the message is about: English Theme." In Mohsen Ghadessy (ed.), *Thematic development in English texts*. London & New York: Pinter. 223–258.

Martin, James R. 2004. "Metafunctional profile of the grammar of Tagalog." In Alice Caffarel, James R. Martin & Christian M.I.M. Matthiessen (eds.), *Language typology: A functional perspective*. Amsterdam: John Benjamins. 255–304.

Martin, James R., Y.J. Doran & Giacomo Figueredo. (eds.). 2019. *Systemic functional language description: Making meaning matter*. Oxon & New York: Routledge.

Martin, James R., Christian M.I.M. Matthiessen & Claire Painter. 2010. *Deploying functional grammar*. Beijing: Commercial Press.

Martin, James R. & Peter R.R. White. 2005. *The language of evaluation: Appraisal in English*. London: Palgrave.

Mathesius, Vilém. 1928. "On linguistic characterology with illustrations from modern English." In *Actes du Premier Congrès International de Linguistes à La Haye, du 10–15 Avril, 1928*. Leiden: A. W. Sijthoff. 56–63.

Mathesius, Vilém. 1975. *A functional analysis of present day English on a general linguistic basis*. Berlin: Mouton de Gruyter.

Matthiessen, Christian M.I.M. 1995a. *Lexicogrammatical cartography: English systems*. Tokyo: International Language Sciences Publishers.

Matthiessen, Christian M.I.M. 1995b. "THEME as an enabling resource in ideational 'knowledge' construction." In Mohsen Ghadessy (ed.), *Thematic development in English texts*. London & New York: Pinter. 20–55.

Matthiessen, Christian M.I.M. 2001. "The environments of translation." In Erich Steiner & Colin Yallop (eds.), *Exploring translation and multilingual text production: Beyond content*. Berlin: Mouton de Gruyter. 41–124.

Matthiessen, Christian M.I.M. 2002. "Combining clauses into clause complexes: A multifaceted view." In Joan L. Bybee & Michael Noonan (eds.), *Complex sentences in grammar and discourse: Essays in honor of Sandra A. Thompson*. Amsterdam & Philadelphia: John Benjamins. 237–322.

Matthiessen, Christian M.I.M. 2009. "Ideas and new directions." In M.A.K. Halliday & Jonathan J. Webster (eds.), *Continuum companion to systemic functional linguistics*. London & New York: Continuum. 12–58.

Matthiessen, Christian M.I.M. 2014a. "Appliable discourse analysis." In Yan Fang & Jonathan J. Webster (eds.), *Developing systemic functional linguistics: Theory and application*. London: Equinox. 135–205.

Matthiessen, Christian M.I.M. 2014b. "Choice in translation: Metafunctional considerations." In Kerstin Kunz, Elke Teich, Silvia Hansen-Schirra, Stella Neumann & Peggy Daut (eds.), *Caught in the middle-language use and translation: A festschrift for Erich Steiner on the occasion of his 60th birthday*. Saarbrücken: Saarland University Press. 271–333.

Matthiessen, Christian M.I.M. 2015a. "English lexicogrammar through text: Text typology and lexicogrammatical patterns." In Xu Xunfeng & Joe Chen (eds.), *Language meaning: Grammar, discourse and corpus*. Shanghai: Shanghai Jiao Tong University Press. 1–49.

Matthiessen, Christian M.I.M. 2015b. "Register in the round: Registerial cartography." *Functional Linguistics* 2(9): 1–48.

Matthiessen, Christian M.I.M. 2015c. "Modelling context and register: The long-term project of registerial cartography." *Letras, Santa Maria* 25(50): 15–90.

Matthiessen, Christian M.I.M. forthcoming. "Translation, multilingual text production and cognition viewed in terms of systemic functional linguistics." manuscript.

Matthiessen, Christian M.I.M., Kazuhiro Teruya & Marvin Lam. 2010. *Key terms in systemic functional linguistics.* London & New York: Continuum.

Matthiessen, Christian M.I.M., Kazuhiro Teruya & Wu Canzhong. 2008. "Multilingual studies as a multi-dimensional space of interconnected language studies." In Jonathan J. Webster (ed.), *Meaning in context: Implementing intelligent applications of language studies.* London & New York: Continuum. 146–220.

Matthiessen, Christian M.I.M., Bo Wang & Yuanyi Ma. 2017a. "Interview with Christian M.I.M. Matthiessen: On translation studies (Part I)." *Linguistics and the Human Sciences* 13(1–2): 201–217.

Matthiessen, Christian M.I.M., Bo Wang & Yuanyi Ma. 2017b. "Interview with Christian M.I.M. Matthiessen: On translation studies (Part II)." *Linguistics and the Human Sciences* 13(3): 339–359.

Matthiessen, Christian M.I.M., Bo Wang & Yuanyi Ma. 2018. "Interview with Christian M.I.M. Matthiessen: On translation studies (Part III)." *Linguistics and the Human Sciences* 14(1): 94–106.

Matthiessen, Christian M.I.M., Bo Wang & Yuanyi Ma. 2019. "Expounding register and registerial cartography in systemic functional linguistics: An interview with Christian M.I.M. Matthiessen." *WORD* 65(2): 93–106.

Mauranen, Anna. 2008. "Universal tendencies in translation." In Gunilla Anderman & Margaret Rogers (eds.), *Incorporating corpora: The linguist and the translator.* Clevedon: Multilingual Matters. 32–48.

Mauranen, Anna & Pekka Kujamäki. (eds.). 2004. *Translation universals: Do they exist?* Amsterdam & Philadelphia: John Benjamins.

Munday, Jeremy. 2001. *Introducing translation studies: Theories and applications.* London & New York: Routledge.

Munday, Jeremy. 2002. "Systems in translation: A systemic model for descriptive translation studies." In Theo Hermans (ed.), *Crosscultural transgressions: Research models in translation studies II: Historical and ideological issues.* Manchester: St Jerome. 76–92.

Munday, Jeremy. 2012. *Evaluation in translation: Critical points of translator decision-making.* London & New York: Routledge.

Munday, Jeremy. 2016. *Introducing translation studies: Theories and applications.* 4th edition. Oxon & New York: Routledge.

Munday, Jeremy. 2018. "A model of appraisal: Spanish interpretations of President Trump's inaugural address 2017." *Perspectives: Studies in Translation Theory and Practice* 26(2): 180–195.

Mwinlaaru, Isaac N. 2018. "Grammaticalising attitude: Clause juncture particles and NEGOTIATION in Dagaare." In Akila Sellami-Baklouti & Lise Fontaine (eds.), *Perspectives from systemic functional linguistics.* Oxon & New York: Routledge. 208–230.

Mwinlaaru, Isaac N. & Winfred Wenhui Xuan. 2016. "A survey of studies in systemic functional language description and typology." *Functional Linguistics* 3(8): 1–41.

Newmark, Peter. 1987. "The use of systemic linguistics in translation analysis and criticism." In Ross Steele & Terry Threadgold (eds.), *Language topics: Essays in honour of Michael Halliday* (volume 1). Amsterdam & Philadelphia: John Benjamins. 293–303.

Newmark, Peter. 1988. *A textbook of translation*. Oxford & New York: Prentice Hall.

Nida, Eugene A. 1964. *Towards a science of translation: With special reference to principles and procedures involved in Bible translating*. Leiden: Brill.

Nida, Eugene A. & Charles R. Taber. 1969. *The theory and practice of translation*. Leiden: Brill.

Pawley, Andrew. 1987. "Encoding events in Kalam and English: Different logics for reporting experience." In Russell S. Tomlin (ed.), *Coherence and grounding in discourse*. Amsterdam & Philadelphia: John Benjamins. 329–361.

Peng, Ling [彭玲]. 2013. 合作原则在《茶馆》翻译中的跨文化应用 [Intercultural application of the cooperative principle in the translation of *Teahouse*]. Master thesis, Soochow University, Suzhou, China.

Pu, Cunxin [濮存昕]. 2007. "用生命拥抱角色 – 常四爷创作体会 [Embrace the character with life: Some experiences on the creation of Master Chang]." In 刘章春 [Liu Zhangchun] (ed.), 《茶馆》的舞台艺术 [Arts of *Teahouse*]. 北京 [Beijing]: 中国戏剧出版社 [China Theatre Press]. 166–171.

Pym, Anthony. 2010. *Exploring translation theories*. London & New York: Routledge.

Ren, Baoxian [任宝贤]. 2007. "《茶馆》点将录 [On the characters in *Teahouse*]." In 刘章春 [Liu Zhangchun] (ed.), 《茶馆》的舞台艺术 [Arts of *Teahouse*]. 北京 [Beijing]: 中国戏剧出版社 [China Theatre Press]. 310–316.

Ren, Xiaofei [任晓霏]. 2008. *登场的译者 – 英若诚戏剧翻译系统研究* [Translator on stage: A systematic study on Ying Ruocheng's drama translation]. 北京 [Beijing]: 中国社会科学出版社 [China Social Sciences Press].

Seuren, Pieter A.M. 1998. *Western linguistics: A historical introduction*. Oxford: Blackwell.

Shen, Linlin [沈琳琳]. 2010. "《茶馆》英译本中文化负载词的翻译策略研究 [Translation strategies on culturally-loaded words in the English version of *Teahouse*]." 海华科技学院学报 [Journal of Huaihai Institute of Technology] 8(8): 72–74.

Shih, Yourong [施佑融]. 2012. 从数来宝到快板书研究 [Study on the evolution from shulaibao to kuaiban storytelling]. Master thesis. National Central University, Taoyuan, Taiwan.

Steiner, Erich. 2002. "Grammatical metaphor in translation—some methods for corpus-based investigations." In Hilde Hasselgard, Stig Johansson, Behrens Bergljot & Cathrine Fabricius-Hansen (eds.), *Information structure in a cross-linguistic perspective*. Amsterdam: Rodopi. 213–228.

Steiner, Erich. 2004. *Translated texts: Properties, variants, evaluations*. Frankfurt am Main: Peter Lang.

Steiner, Erich. 2005. "Halliday and translation theory: Enhancing the options, broadening the range, and keeping the ground." In Ruqaiya Hasan, Christian M.I.M. Matthiessen & Jonathan J. Webster (eds.), *Continuing discourse on language: A functional perspective* (volume 1). London: Equinox. 481–500.

Steiner, Erich. 2008. "Explicitation: Towards an empirical and corpus-based methodology." In Jonathan J. Webster (eds.), *Meaning in context: Implementing intelligent applications of language studies*. London & New York: Continuum. 234–277.

Steiner, Erich. 2015. "Halliday's contribution to a theory of translation." In Jonathan J. Webster (ed.), *The Bloomsbury companion to M.A.K. Halliday*. London & New York: Bloomsbury. 412–426.

Steiner, Erich. 2017. "Methodological cross-fertilization: Empirical methodologies in (computational) linguistics and translation studies." In Oliver Czulo & Silvia Hansen-Schirra (eds.), *Crossroads between contrastive linguistics, translation studies and machine translation*. Berlin: Language Science Press. 65–90.

Steiner, Erich. 2019. "Theorizing and modelling translation." In Geoff Thompson, Wendy L. Bowcher, Lise Fontaine & David Schönthal (eds.), *The Cambridge handbook of systemic functional linguistics*. Cambridge: Cambridge University Press.

Steiner, Erich & Colin Yallop. (eds.). 2001. *Exploring translation and multilingual text production*. Berlin: Mouton de Gruyter.

Tam, Kwok-kan [谭国根]. 2004. "前言:《茶馆》中苦涩的幽默与历史视野 [Introduction: Lao She's bitter humour and historical re-visioning in *Teahouse*]." In 老舍 [Lao She], 茶馆 [Teahouse]. 香港 [Hong Kong]: Chinese University Press. ix–xlix.

Taylor, Christopher. 1993. "Systemic linguistics and translation." *Occasional Papers in Systemic Linguistics* 7: 87–103.

Teich, Elke. 2001. "Towards a model for the description of cross-linguistic divergence and commonality in translation." In Erich Steiner & Colin Yallop (eds.), *Exploring translation and multilingual text production: Beyond content*. Berlin: Mouton de Gruyter. 41–124.

Teich, Elke. 2003. *Cross-linguistic variation in system and text: A methodology for the investigation of translations and comparable texts*. Berlin & New York: Mouton de Gruyter.

Teruya, Kazuhiro. 2004. "Metafunctional profile of the grammar of Japanese." In Alice Caffarel, James R. Martin & Christian M.I.M. Matthiessen (eds.), *Language typology: A functional perspective*. Amsterdam: John Benjamins. 185–254.

Teruya, Kazuhiro. 2007. *A systemic functional grammar of Japanese* (volume 1 & 2). London & New York: Continuum.

Tong, Chao [童超]. 2007. "庞太监创造过程追记 [A retrospective note on the creative process of Eunuch Pang]." In 刘章春 [Liu Zhangchun] (ed.), 《茶馆》的舞台艺术 [Arts of *Teahouse*]. 北京 [Beijing]: 中国戏剧出版社 [China Theatre Press]. 106–113.

Toury, Gideon. 2004. "Probabilistic explanations in translation studies: Welcome as they are, would they qualify as universals?." In Anna Mauranen & Pekka Kujamäki (eds.), *Translation universals: Do they exist?* Amsterdam: John Benjamins. 15–32.

Ventola, Eija. 1995. "Thematic development and translation." In Mohsen Ghadessy (ed.), *Thematic development in English texts*. London & New York: Pinter. 85–104.

Vince, Ronald W. 2010. "Monologue." In Dennis Kennedy (ed.), *The Oxford companion to theatre and performance*. Oxford: Oxford University Press. 402.

Wang, Bo. 2014. "Theme in translation: A systemic functional linguistic perspective." *International Journal of Comparative Literature & Translation Studies* 2(4): 54–63.

Wang, Bo. 2017. *Lao She's Cha Guan (Teahouse) and its English translations: A systemic functional perspective on drama translation*. Doctoral thesis, the Hong Kong Polytechnic University, Hong Kong.

Wang, Bo [王博] & Yuanyi Ma [马园艺]. 2016. "译者的选择 – 《茶馆》粤语译本的翻译策略 [Choice of the translator: Translation strategies for the Cantonese version of *Teahouse*]." In 杨连瑞 [Yang Lianrui] (ed.), *Foreign language research in China: 2015*. 青岛 [Qingdao]: 中国海洋大学出版社 [China Ocean University Press]. 82–92.

Wang, Bo & Yuanyi Ma. 2018. "Textual and logical choices in the translations of dramatic monologue in *Teahouse*." In Akila Sellami-Baklouti & Lise Fontaine (eds.), *Perspectives from systemic functional linguistics*. Oxon & New York: Routledge. 140–162.

Wang, Bo & Yuanyi Ma. 2019. "The recreation of Pock-Mark Liu and Wang Lifa in two Chinese translations of *Teahouse*: A systemic functional analysis of mood choices." In Kumaran Rajandran & Shakila A. Manan (eds.), *Discourse of South East Asia*. Singapore: Springer. 189–208.

Wang, Bo & Yuanyi Ma. in press. *Systemic functional translation studies: Theoretical insights and new directions*. Sheffield: Equinox.

Whittaker, Rachel. 1995. "Theme, processes and the realization of meanings in academic articles." In Mohsen Ghadessy (ed.), *Thematic development in English texts*. London & New York: Pinter. 105–128.

Yang, Lixin [杨立新]. 2007. "回头看《茶馆》排练 [Look back on the rehearsal of *Teahouse*]." In 刘章春 [Liu Zhangchun] (ed.), 《茶馆》的舞台艺术 [Arts of *Teahouse*]. 北京 [Beijing]: 中国戏剧出版社 [China Theatre Press]. 172–179.

Yang, Yichen. 2016. *Performability and translation: A case study of the production and reception of Ying Ruocheng's translations*. Ph.D. thesis, Lingnan University, Hong Kong.

Ying, Ruocheng [英若诚]. 1999. "序言 [Preface]." In 老舍 [Lao She], 茶馆 [Teahouse]. 北京 [Beijing]: 中国对外翻译出版公司 [China Translation and Publishing Corporation]. 1–11.

Ying, Ruocheng [英若诚]. 2007. "重演《茶馆》的一些感想 [Some thoughts on restaging *Teahouse*]." In 刘章春 [Liu Zhangchun] (ed.), 《茶馆》的舞台艺术 [Arts of *Teahouse*]. 北京 [Beijing]: 中国戏剧出版社 [China Theatre Press]. 100–105.

Ying, Ruocheng & Claire Conceison. 2009. *Voices carry: Behind bars and backstage during China's revolution and reform*. Lanham: Roman & Littlefield.

Yu, Hailing & Wu Canzhong. 2016. "Recreating the image of Chan master Huineng: The roles of MOOD and MODALITY." *Functional Linguistics* 3(4): 1–21.

Yu, Hailing & Wu Canzhong. 2017. "Recreating the image of Chan master Huineng: The role of personal pronouns." *Target* 29(1): 64–86.

Yu, Shizhi [于是之]. 2007. "演王利发小记 [Notes on performing Wang Lifa]." In 刘章春 [Liu Zhangchun] (ed.), 《茶馆》的舞台艺术 [Arts of *Teahouse*]. 北京 [Beijing]: 中国戏剧出版社 [China Theatre Press]. 76–81.

Zhang, Fuyuan [张福元]. 2008. "活得最明白的人 [The man who lives a most self-conscious life]." In 刘章春 [Liu Zhangchun] (ed.), 《茶馆》在世界 [*Teahouse* in the world]. 北京 [Beijing]: 中国戏剧出版社 [China Theatre Press]. 274–275.

Zhang, Guixing [张桂兴]. 2000. 老舍资料考释 [Explanations of materials on Lao She]. 北京 [Beijing]: 中国国际广播出版社 [China International Broadcasting Press].

Zheng, Rong [郑榕]. 1983. "《茶馆》的艺术感染力 [The aesthetic appeal of *Teahouse*]." In Uwe Kräuter (ed.), 东方舞台上的奇迹 – 《茶馆》在西欧 [A miracle on the oriental stage: *Teahouse* in West Europe]. 北京 [Beijing]: 文化艺术出版社 [Culture and Art Publishing House]. 153–175.

Zheng, Rong [郑榕]. 2007. "扮演常四爷的一点体会 [Some thoughts on acting Master Chang]." In 刘章春 [Liu Zhangchun] (ed.), 《茶馆》的舞台艺术 [Arts of *Teahouse*]. 北京 [Beijing]: 中国戏剧出版社 [China Theatre Press]. 82–87.

Zhu, Chunshen. 1996. "From functional grammar and speech act theory to structure of meaning: A three-dimensional perspective on translating." *Meta* 41(3): 338–355.

Index

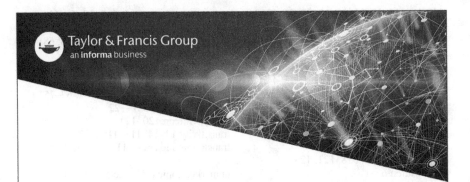

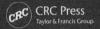

Printed in the United States
by Baker & Taylor Publisher Services

Printed in the United States
by Baker & Taylor Publisher Services